D1557372

"FAR BETTER is it to dare things, to win glorious triumphs, even though checkered by failure...than to rank with those poor spirits who neither enjoy nor suffer much, because they live in a gray twilight that knows not victory nor defeat."

"It is not the critic who counts; not the man who points out how the strong man stumbles, or where the doer of deeds could have done them better. The credit belongs to the man who is actually in the arena, whose face is marred by dust and sweat and blood; who strives valiantly; who errs, who comes short again and again, because there is no effort without error and shortcoming, but who does actually strive to do the deeds, who knows great enthusiasms, the great devotions, who spends himself in a worthy cause; who at the best knows in the end the triumph of high achievement, and who at the worst, if he fails, at least fails while daring greatly, so that his place shall never be with those cold and timid souls who neither know victory nor defeat."

— *Theodore Roosevelt*

These words inspired Rob and he lived by them every day.

MAN
WITH A
BACKPACK

One Regular Guy's Fight Against Stomach Cancer

ROB LUKENS
REBECCA LUKENS

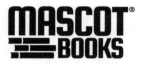

www.mascotbooks.com

Man With A Backpack:
One Regular Guy's Fight Against Stomach Cancer

Family Portrait Provided by Sue Reno Portraits

For more information, please contact:
Mascot Books
560 Herndon Parkway #120
Herndon, VA 20170
info@mascotbooks.com

Library of Congress Control Number: 2016910407

CPSIA Code: PBANG0816A
ISBN-13: 978-1-63177-570-3

Printed in the United States

This book is dedicated to Rob's children, Abbie and Finn. They are two of the strongest and most courageous kids I know. May we continue to heal together but never forget how fortunate we were to have had such an amazing father and husband. I love you both so much.

Mom

NO ST◦MACH FOR CANCER®

Supporting Research. Empowering Families.

ACKNOWLEDGMENTS

I would like to thank all of those who have given their support over the past few years. The outpouring of prayers and emotional and monetary support has been overwhelming, and we will always be forever grateful.

A special thank you to Wil, Rob's brother. Because of his encouragement, hours of time, and emotional support, I was able to have the strength to see this book through for Rob, allowing me to share the stinging reality of cancer that unfortunately so many are faced with.

This book depicts the actual and true events of Rob's battle with cancer. The goal was not to offend anyone in any way by the things he wrote but to give a complete, raw perspective of the reality of cancer and the ripple effects it has.

Gastric cancer is currently the third leading cause of death from cancer worldwide with one million new cases diagnosed each year. Please support early diagnosis and prevention of stomach cancer by making a donation to No Stomach For Cancer®. Doing so will help raise awareness and support research. www.nostomachforcancer.org

CONTENTS

CHAPTER ONE
The Day I Will Never Forget

Fred Shero (1925-1990)

Beloved coach of the Philadelphia Flyers in the 1970s. He led the team known as the "Broad Street Bullies" to two Stanley Cups in 1974 and 1975 and later died from stomach cancer.

This chapter is a visceral introduction to the process of learning you have cancer, telling people about it, and the first things one does to deal with it.

WHAT would you do if you were suddenly told that you had cancer? At age 40, you may be sailing through life, worrying about the big meeting at work next week, thinking about the sports your kids will play this fall or your next vacation plans. Then, your entire world is turned upside down, completely. And it is not just any cancer. It's stomach cancer, which is a particularly nasty and deadly variety. You are probably thinking that this will never happen to you. And that's what I thought, until Monday, July 22, 2013, when it happened to me.

In the mid-morning of July 22, 2013, I arrived at a tan, stuccoed, low-rise office building on the edge of my hometown of West Chester, Pennsylvania. The building housed a Gastrointestinal Center, and I was there for a routine endoscopy.

Becky, my wife, and kids (Abbie, then age nine, and Finn, then age six) dropped me off, thinking this would be a quick and routine visit. She took the kids to the pool, and I disappeared behind the doors to start my procedure. I checked into the office, surrounded by other patients, and went off on a stretcher to get my Propofol. "Milk of Amnesia," I've heard some anesthesiologists call it.

I had complained of stomach pain for months now but nothing helped. We all thought that this would be a routine procedure, as my health was impeccable. I was a strong 170-pound, forty-year-old man with pretty impressive muscle tone and a full head of hair.

They wheeled me back to a sterile room. As the Propofol went in, I quickly went to sleep. The doctor sent an endoscope—a video camera—down my esophagus to take a look. We all thought that the camera would snap a few photos of an ulcer or grab a sample of something benign for a pathology report.

Instead, as my fuzzy drug-induced vision slowly came into focus, the doctor showed me a strange picture. I expected to see an ulcer or something, but this looked nothing like anything I could have imagined.

Shit! That doesn't look good at all, I thought, as I stared at a mangled and messy tangle of flesh and blood. It was not the kind of thing you could just pop out with a sharp knife and get on with things. Like cancer flashcards, he showed me a mass of tumors that took up the entire picture from side to side.

Immediately, I reached out to my bride, my wife Becky of nearly twelve years. Here are the texts that flew between us:

Rob: I'm done—r u here? They are about to tell me what's up if you want to come back w/o the kids I presume. If not that's ok.

(I didn't want to alarm her via text!)

Becky: I'm on my way - kids r in the car

Becky: I'm only still in town driving

Rob: Ok - then just take your time. No rush.

Becky: Do u want me to leave them in the car a second while I come in? There in about 5 minutes.

Rob: No - bring them into the waiting room. Stay there until I come out. In on the third floor of the b building.

Becky: Do they want me in there when they tell u?

Becky: Finn has no shirt - not sure what to do - we just parked.

Rob: Just come in - they want you to come back.

Becky: I'm here out in the waiting room.

Becky: Everything ok now I'm freaking out

So it all started very mundanely. She came in, and we saw the pictures together. We cried, and our bodies shook with terror in the sterile, starkly decorated exam room that reeked of rubbing alcohol and latex.

The doctor told me it looked like cancer, and they would have to do other tests to make sure. We cried more and then had to exit through the waiting room to face the kids with a straight face. I was scared to leave the room because I knew we needed to pull ourselves together somehow, and I was a mess. My face was beet red and my eyes were uncontrollably watery.

Becky's perspective on this initial shock is a little different. She left the kids in the waiting room and immediately saw the nurses whispering about her. She saw me sobbing with a box of tissues and still didn't know why. She didn't cry but was in a state of shock. The nurses assumed she knew what had happened. They gently wrapped her in a warm blanket, handed her a box of tissues, and tried to console her before she even knew what was going on. All she wanted to do was throw that box of tissues in the face of the nurse. Shock set in deeply, and we cried together.

We left the room and entered the short hallway. Just outside of the door, there was a couple I recognized. I didn't even say "hi," but kept my head down and kept walking. Did they hear all of the sobbing? Were they able to overhear all of the questions? I sure hoped they did not because I would hate to think that they, people I barely knew, actually found out about this before anyone else. Later, I found out they were going through something major too—perhaps they found out even at that same moment.

Either way, we both felt the same thing, and Becky summed it up perfectly later, saying, "Our lives were changed on the day we were given the diagnosis. Everything that we thought was important or that we worried about now seemed stupid." She continued, "Everything seemed pointless."

We left the office building on a warm day with the sun seemingly extra-bright, as if to tease us. I broke down in the blood lab where we stopped on the way home. Just fifteen minutes after I found all of this out, there I was, sobbing in front of complete strangers. The lab workers in their white coats tried to console me.

"You'll be fine," they said mechanically. The phlebotomist went through her entire life history as a feeble attempt to offer consolation. The story oddly ended with her lover getting dementia at age 45, which was tragic and completely unrelated.

I soon found out that this is the normal reaction that people have when they encounter someone like me—a victim of cancer. It is an awful, knee-jerk reaction. People co-opt the other's illness in the midst of conversation and insert their own situation, usually without anything productive coming of it.

The worst part is they are not even aware they're doing it, so it is hard to get mad at them. People are scared of cancer, even when they don't have it. This is one of the Top 10 crimes against cancer patients; probably near the top.

We drove home slowly from the lab. Our home was just a few miles away on the other side of town. I decided that there would be no more work for me that day. When we arrived home, we were simply stunned and sat in silence. Tears welled in our eyes as the kids ran off to play in another part of the house. Their gleeful laughs did not sync with the news we just heard.

Looking around the house, my mind started to spin. I spotted the dog and seethed with anger when I realized that this damn, half-blind dog of ours, our German short-haired pointer, Hudson, would probably live longer than me. When I passed the twin goldfish, Lickety and Split, the same thought ran through my mind. *Those damn fish might still be swimming in that tank when I'm dead! They could all outlive me.*

About an hour later, reality clicked in, and I started calculating what to do next and thought through all of the what-ifs. I set up an appointment with an oncologist. I spoke to my primary doctor. I wanted to get things moving here.

And then I became obsessed with numbers. Sitting on the couch, I fumbled through records and searched through the Internet for all of our bank accounts, mutual funds, retirement, and of course, life insurance. As it turns out, our life insurance was totally inadequate. *Damn, why didn't I double that? Triple it? What will Becky do when I'm dead?* This all immediately ran through my mind like ticker tape.

I continued to spend the next couple of days frantically calculating numbers to see how it would all play out if I died. I called Social Security and got two completely different answers about monthly payouts if I croaked.

"This is important!" I tried to tell the Social Security officers. "I have just been given a possible death sentence, and I need to know this stuff and know that it's right!" I exclaimed.

While worrying about the cash situation, I simultaneously went to the place that I shouldn't have: the Internet. I tried to resist the urge.

"Don't Google it, Rob. Don't do it!" I screamed in my head.

But, oh, I couldn't resist, and I'd dare anyone in the same situation to admit that they could resist too.

I Googled "stomach cancer," and it looked like I might have a 50/50 chance of survival. I later discovered that this 50/50 figure is a little too generous, and it is kind of fluid depending on who you ask and what stage you're in. Early on, this death rate filled my head every second of every day.

Then I just sat down on our pilled golden couch and waited for a while. The show *Ellen* was on in the background while a stream of thoughts ran through my head.

I have to tell my mom, I thought. *I have to tell the kids.*

Shit, everyone I know is going to freak out! Will I be treated normal at all once they know? Will I be alive to see the MLB game advertised on TV? And meanwhile, I've got to figure out a way for my wife to be financially self-sufficient. All of this occurred in the two hours since my death sentence.

As I sat there, alone, on that same couch, I had to mentally grapple with some other realities. *How much does a casket cost anyway? A funeral? A grave plot? It seems like a slap in the face,* I think at about minute 120. A loved one dies, and then you have to feed people and pay for embalming and all of that craziness. It should be the other way around. When you need it the most at a funeral, the invitees should all pay for these services when you die. When you have a birthday, a baby, a marriage, and you're already happy, people pay you!

Wednesday, July 24th was a big day. It was two days after the initial shock, and I got my blood results and biopsy results, and had a CAT scan done, which would show if I was riddled with tumors or not. For some reason, it already seemed mechanical—going to the hospital for the CAT scan with iodine contrast and thinking about the results.

Luckily, I figured out a psychological approach to this, which is not altogether foreign to me. Like all of the good leadership books I read, I needed to acknowledge the adversity—identify it like a WWII general, not ignore it—and then optimistically decide that I'm going to beat it using the resources available to me. I would later realize how difficult it is to think this way throughout all of the challenges and negative forces pulling me downward. The further along I went in this battle against cancer, the harder it was to stay chipper and full of enthusiasm for beating it forever. Actually, it was impossible. This challenge was fundamentally different than anything I'd ever come across.

On the day I learned *for sure* that I had the "C" word, it was Christmas in July. It was a nice early Christmas present on July 25, 2013. It figured that I would probably reemerge from all of this—the chemo, the surgery, the recovery, the radiation—in some form around the real Christmas, so I guess that was pretty fitting.

I was wrong—*so* wrong, as it turned out—about the timing. It would end up being a much longer ordeal than I could have ever imagined, lasting at least another year—a lifetime, actually.

The official news came from a phone call. "Mr. Lukens, I'm very sorry but the biopsy shows that you do have stomach cancer."

While I was at work, Becky was muddling around the house trying to keep herself busy. *This isn't supposed to happen to us; we are too young. This is for old people,* she thought. *What about growing old together watching our kids grow up?* she asked herself. *What about enjoying life, getting gray hair together or losing it together, and becoming grandparents?*

These thoughts are like poison and have turned our lives as we know them upside down. She waited for that same phone call that I had just gotten on my cell. When she received it, she was in shock. She collapsed in our cold, dark basement in disbelief. She sat shaking and crying and saying over and over again, "No, no, no!"

She sat motionless on that dusty old couch, that same couch we have had since we first got married. All the memories on that couch, all the stories came flooding through her mind: the laughs, holding our babies for the first time, and now being told that her husband has cancer for the first time. Now every time she goes down to the basement and looks at that couch, that is all she can think about, that day in July, a day she'd like to erase from her memory.

I was still at work after the official cancer notification. I calmly wrapped up my conversation with my business manager. We were talking about moving some funds around to cover checks while she was on vacation. I was stoic and calm.

Becky called in the middle of the meeting, and she was frantic. The doctor had told her through a similar, impersonal phone call at home. When I got home, she was sobbing and shaking in the basement of the house, still clutching the phone.

This was the same day they announced the birth of Kate and Prince William's baby, a prince, who we later learned was named George. That was the day I learned of all of this—July 25, 2014, Christmas in July.

As Becky said it best, "When the whole world was waiting the arrival of the new prince of England, bringing the motherland a wonderful 'Christmas in July' gift, we were delivered cancer at our home."

When I got home I met her in the basement, where she still lay crying. Eventually, we moved upstairs. The kids were in their rooms, so it was just her and me witnessing and enacting this seminal moment of our lives with the half-blind dog to witness.

I started babbling. I said we would beat this, we would win, and we would kick this thing's ass. I told her cancer didn't know that it picked the wrong guy to mess with and that we had over a thousand friends that would pull for us, protect us, and nurture us.

As we stood there, swaying and sobbing in the kitchen, I said, "This is big news. A lot of people will be stunned." I told her, "I don't want people to look at me differently."

How awkward it would be for people to talk to someone who had just been diagnosed with cancer! Did you bring up small talk, the weather, the Phillies' pitching, and whatnot, or just cut to the chase and deal with it head-on? I would find all of this out. And if you deal with it head on, is it with a sober somber, "Sorry, dude," or something a little more cheery like, "Rob, you're going to kick that cancer's ass!"

I would later find out that cancer pretty much dominated all conversations for the next year and beyond. I couldn't help it—people would ask about it, and I would go on about my chemo or radiation or diet or scheduling surgeries or procedures. TMI—too much information—most likely in most conversational cases. But I didn't care because I was the one with cancer, dammit, and I would tell people the truth about their questions. People would feel obligated to ask, and the ones who didn't seemed insensitive, even though they were probably just too nervous to bring it up.

All of this was swimming through my head while I still gripped my wife tightly on that late morning, in the kitchen, on Christmas in July.

Then, all kinds of stupid stuff came flowing out of my mouth. I wanted, no, I demanded, that everyone who knew and loved me send me a baseball cap to wear for support when I went bald. It would be a rainbow of teams, vacation spots, stupid sayings, universities, and brand names. I planned to take it all and wear them with pride—even New York teams, if someone sent one.

In fact, I said we would start a new charity called "Caps for Cancer Dads," and become famous! We would go on the *Today Show* to talk about it. "It's going to be fantastic. Oh, and by the way, I will live through this," I told her confidently then. Nearly two years later, the hats sit in a pile on my closet floor, forgotten like that initial rush of enthusiasm.

Later, in solitude, my mind jumped to a game plan. *I need a five year plan*, I thought. It looked like they measured things in five years for cancer survivors, so I wanted to be part of that 28 percent that made it. When I looked a little more closely at the stats, it was really more like a 28-percent than 50-percent survival rate.

I found out this grim survival rate in a very casual fashion. When I met with my oncologist, she charted out my treatment plan like an NFL coach. She passed me a handful of papers that documented why this particular treatment of chemo before surgery made sense. It was an explanation of the study, ironically called the "Magic Study," which outlined the chemo before surgery stats. The fine print, near the end, showed the results of this study. They considered this 28-percent survival rate a success. *Wow, if that's success, then what's a failure? Sure death?*

So, my statistics are about 28 percent that I'll live past the five-year mark, which would be the year 2018. I decided that I had a 50/50 chance because I was young. I was pissed and determined when I discovered this survival rate in the silence of my own home after our visit to the doctor. That was my own personal, amateur assessment, but I believed it. It seemed like a nice even number, and I thought to myself, *That's not bad. I can deal with those odds.* I wanted to see my daughter and son graduate from high school and college and get married, dammit.

I've never been super-competitive, and that's one of my weaknesses. I've never had any cutthroat, "eye of the tiger" killer instinct, but I've always had lots of just straight determination. I would have been a good long distance runner if I had been encouraged to do that at a younger age. Now I needed both resolve and complete and utter competitive spirit. My goal: Make it past that five-year mark and outlive the dog...or at least those damn goldfish, Lickety and Split.

Being a linear analytical thinker, I broke my tasks down to three primarily: *With my wife, even though I hope I'm here, I need to make sure she has to worry as little as possible if I'm gone. I need to literally set her up for success. Perhaps even job training so she can live without me? I could use my connections to get her a job now or later? The other approach is to accumulate more money, but it would be hard to accumulate enough to make it so she didn't have to work?* The second role, loving and supporting her, was a given, but I needed to leave this world knowing that she was okay if I was going to be checking out, which I didn't plan on doing. But with anything, small or serious, I always need to know the plan B or C in any scenario. With my kids, my third role, I would strive to provide them with a normal, loving five-plus years and more fatherly attention. And if I could add a fourth, regarding my work, it would be to ensure the success of my institution, which would help keep my job and benefits along the way.

Money

The money was the worst part. Within minutes of learning that I probably had cancer, I immediately assessed the worst-case scenario. What would happen to my wife and kids if I died? How would they live and keep this house? The answer was that it wouldn't be easy.

The second worst part was the more self-deprecating question that always followed these internal queries: *How could I be so stupid?* This ran through my head most days and did for the next two years. If I had only taken out a simple million-dollar policy, half of my worries would be gone. She could live off the interest and social security. Heck, she could even buy a beach house for her and the kids if she wanted. She wouldn't feel compelled to remarry unless she really wanted to. It would have been so easy. Ah, hindsight.

So I started developing a plan—multiple plans, actually—for how they could live without me. *I'm damaged goods, forever, and no life insurance company would ever return my phone calls. So I must seek other ways to raise money and build income for us while I'm alive, and for her when I'm dead.*

I thought about this daily. *What will she do when I'm gone?* I'd always been the breadwinner and she the one who juggled her own design business, while handling most of the household and kids' needs.

In order to get a full handle on this, I had to run several calculations. First, how much did it cost for me to be alive? I did a quick check on my personal costs of living: cell phone, car, car insurance, gas, portion of health insurance, food, entertainment and lunches out, etc. I sadly discovered that I, as a single part of this family, once removed, would save very little money. It was the family unit that cost the most, and the individual parts (us individually) provided little or no savings once removed. The mortgage, utilities, Becky's nicer family car, and everything else would all cost the same. In very rare areas our expenses might go down by a quarter, but the overall picture was more like 10 percent savings from me not being on the planet.

I need to bitch about this for a while. There are way too many economies of scale worked into a family's expenses. There are really very little savings when one quarter of the equation is removed. Even if it's the most high maintenance person! Think about it. The mortgage would be the same (and she needs to keep this house!), family health insurance policies are the same, the utilities are the same, and even the damn YMCA membership is the same. The only net gain is less food eaten, which I can barely eat after my surgery anyway, less wine and beer consumed, cheaper dinners out, loss of one paid-off car, and maybe a few medical expenses saved. This saddened me, as I wished my death could provide a steeper family discount.

I actually spent almost my entire first full day being cancer-aware on the phone with Social Security. *How much would she really get?* I wanted to know. I was on hold for forty-five minutes the first time, and the lady didn't seem to get the importance of this to me. *This is critical, not hypothetical,* I thought. I need to know how much money my wife will get if I'm dead. The Social Security representative initially said she'd get a low amount "split three ways," and I freaked.

"Split three ways!" I exclaimed. "On my official sheet of paper—you know, those green and white ones you get once a year—it says that I get more than double that!"

"Hold please," she said as she checked for another ten minutes. "Sir, I have just reconfirmed, it is split *three* ways." She emphasized the *three* and made it sound menacingly final.

I hung up the phone, poked around on the Internet and found what I wanted: a copy of that green and white sheet. I called back and was on hold for one hour this time before I was disconnected.

I called back again, waited a half-hour, and then talked to a nice woman who said, "*No,* that's that original number per person, so each child and your wife would get that subject to a much larger limit."

Bingo! This literally made my day, that first day. On the day that I learned of my cancer, I was genuinely happy and felt that my persistence paid off. So here's what I came up with: With Social Security payments and me out of the picture, Becky would still need health insurance and a steady part time job, but could likely stay in the house.

Gathering Evidence

My other most immediate instinct in that first week was to gather evidence. I needed to know about people who had died at age 40, or close to it. I quietly and sneakily planted myself in a part of the house with some privacy and pulled out my smartphone. I used the Internet for this quackery research, and after viewing that list, I immediately skipped it because I didn't plan on being in it.

Instead, I moved on to famous people who were diagnosed with something horrible around this age but beat it. *That's a better thought*, I decided. People like Lance Armstrong, Mario Lemieux, and Sheryl Crow filled this list. Closer to home, I knew of a friend who kicked an aggressive case of breast cancer.

Through some more surreptitious online searches, it seems like age 39 is the last year that you are considered a "young" cancer patient. Another reason why, at age 40, I guess I'm screwed. Here are a few "young" ones who popped up on my screen:

- Christina Applegate contracted breast cancer at age 39.

- Ethan Zahn, winner of Survivor Africa, Stage 2 Hodgkin's Disease.

- Ryan Buell, of A&E's *Paranormal State*, which I had never heard of, was just diagnosed with pancreatic cancer at age 30. Now that's a really bad diagnosis.

But it was difficult to find celebrities or sports stars that beat stomach cancer. Heck, each year in the U.S., only 22,000 people are diagnosed with it, and about half of that die every year. That diagnosis rate is compared to the nearly 200,000 breast cancer patients and 240,000 prostate cancer victims. So stomach cancer is way down on the priority list as far as public attention is concerned, and I needed to dig a little deeper or allow other data in to my analysis. To do that, I turned to history.

If you go onto Ranker.com, it will list literally hundreds of people over history that have died from stomach cancer, or any other malady that you choose to filter your results. It's pretty macabre, actually, but worked for me, giving me a full-blown, depressing catalog of 234 people. They were listed in alphabetical order, and the first ones I recognized were Edsel Ford, born in 1893, and John Ford, born 1894. This did not comfort me at all.

But later in the Ranker.com list were some interesting finds. Among those killed by my own cancer was Fred Rogers, Mr. Rogers from *Mr. Rogers*. The list also included John Wayne, Liz Claiborne, and Napoleon Bonaparte (so that's why he was holding his abdomen all the time?).

Patrick Henry ("Give me liberty, or give me death!") and Roy Disney also populated the list, along with authors Gertrude Stein and Tom Clancy. All of these illustrious figures died from stomach cancer.

Let's look a little closer at some of these. Liz Claiborne, for instance, lived about ten years *after* her initial diagnosis. *I'll consider that a huge success. That would get me to fifty years old, which is plenty of time.* She was diagnosed in 1997 with a "rare form of cancer that affects the lining of the stomach" and then died in 2007. She was seventy-seven years old. *Again, if Liz can do that at seventy-seven, then I can make it at least ten years now. I'd be pretty happy with that.*

I shuffled in my secret spot, near the back of the house where Becky couldn't find me, and continued my quest. After searching a little more and finding few victims I connected to...Bingo! I found my man. It was Fred Shero. Darn, my dad would be proud if I was compared to him. He was the coach of the Philadelphia Flyers during their two-year Stanley Cup run in the 1970s.

Mr. Shero was diagnosed in 1982, but died in 1990. That was a good eight years. In the 1980s, which might as well have been the dark ages of medicine, he made it an extra eight years in his fifties. I could certainly make it ten, then, as a forty-year-old. *I'll consider Shero a success story as well.*

I'm so disappointed in myself. I'm so anti-Wikipedia, and here I am, relying on it as if it's the Bible. Oh well, they say cancer changes you, and there is no written encyclopedia of stomach cancer victims.

The next question that popped into my head was: What did Fred Shero do during those eight years of his diagnosis? I had to know. So I picked up the phone and tried to track down his family, but I didn't get too far. His son, Ray, was then the General Manager for the Pittsburgh Penguins, and hard to get in touch with. In fact, Fred Shero was elected to the Hockey Hall of Fame just a few weeks before my diagnosis. I was determined to contact Ray to find out how his father did with the disease and what he did with those last eight years. I reached out to his son by sending a heartfelt letter to him at the Penguins front office, but he didn't reply.

I wanted to try again, realizing that Ray would have only been twenty when his father was diagnosed, and twenty-eight when his father died. I felt some kind of shallow camaraderie, as I was only twenty-one when my father was diagnosed with cancer, and was twenty-four when he died. But this quest to get his attention was the middle of the 2013 Playoffs, and the Penguins were going deep. So I thought I'd hold off until the off-season.

I later reached out to Ed Snider, Flyers owner since the 1960s, at his home and work address with similar questions, thinking that a Philly man might respond somehow. I asked if I could contact the Shero family, how Fred did during his diagnosis, and why Flyers Charities didn't do anything for stomach cancer organizations, which killed one of their greats. Unfortunately, I never received a response.

I gave up on the Internet for the time being and forgot about my quest to find like situations for several days until I heard from a friend. Sitting at my desk at work, through an email from that friend, I found the Holy Grail of stomach cancer survivors. I found him mostly by accident and certainly without Google. It was John Hope Franklin. He is among the most famous historians of all time and pioneered the field of African American History. Thanks to my advisor at Temple University, I now know that John Hope Franklin was a stomach cancer survivor. According to my doctoral advisor in History at Temple University:

> "My teacher and friend, John Hope Franklin, had an operation for stomach cancer in 1987 when he was seventy-one years old. Six months later, he made a trip to Germany where he visited me in Goettingen, where I was teaching as a Fulbright Professor. I was astounded to see that he was completely recovered, hale and hearty, his voice strong and sonorous as ever. He returned that fall to Duke University (where, though emeritus, he by his own choice taught one course), continued to write and lecture until he passed on in 2009 at age 93."

So John Hope Franklin, one of the best historians of all time who pioneered all and every aspect of African American History and Studies, lived for another twenty-two years after being diagnosed at age 71! Another twenty-two years would get me to sixty-two, which I would be thrilled about. Just think about what I could do with another *twenty-two years*! I could accumulate more wealth to help my family and be happy with them instead of just counting off the days. I could publish books, have an impact, see a grandchild or two, watch my kids grow up and go through college. Another twenty-two years would put Finn at twenty-eight years old, and Abbie at thirty-one. That would be plenty. *Now I'm going to wish for JHF's twenty-two years.* I would squeeze a hell of a lot into those years. Each day would be packed full of life, love, and other remarkable stuff.

Later I would realize how hard this was in my post-operative state, as I diminished away through early 2015, losing weight and strength, and feeling more and more pain. *Man, my body is messed up. I can barely get off the couch now. Why? The surgery, the chemo, and the proton therapy have taken a huge toll.* Again, the ordeal went well beyond just simple treatment and surgery. Recovery from all of this proved to be the most difficult part, and it dragged on for years.

I quickly went off to the library and found John Hope Franklin's autobiography, *Mirror to America*. I rushed home and for a night or two I read—no, scoured—the entire book for this seminal cancer moment in this man's life. I wanted to find out what Dr. Franklin experienced, when he discovered he had this same awful cancer that now rocked my world, even though there was a big age difference. What kind of treatment and surgery did he endure? What was his philosophy for beating this evil menace?

After pouring over his *Mirror to America*, what I found was, out of nearly 400 pages of his book, Franklin dedicated two small paragraphs to the illness that now overwhelmed my entire life story. It appeared that this seventy-one-year-old man was merely inconvenienced by this diagnosis that cramped his style for a short while in 1987.

Dr. Franklin had surgery and then after completed "painless chemotherapy and, in due course, resumed my normal activities." (p. 315) *"Resumed my normal activities!" Am I making too big a deal about this?* Here's a guy who was seventy-one, could have thrown in the towel and had already lived a full, wonderful life full of amazing things. And he was simply inconvenienced by this diagnosis, surgery, and therapy! John Hope—my hero! *Oh, I hope I live another twenty-two years. Just get me to sixty-two.*

Still within the first week of diagnosis, I ruminated over Lance Armstrong late one night at home in front of the TV during a sleepless night. *I don't care about the doping thing, unless that actually helped him beat cancer—in which case, where do I sign up? What I do care about is that he beat it; he beat it somehow.* I was just about to get his book, *It's Not About the Bike,* or something like that, and see what his secrets were. I went onto Livestrong—the cancer website for his nonprofit organization by the same name—to see what it was all about and glean some key guiding information about how to "win" this.

But then I paused and thought, *Wait, do I really need some pseudo sports celebrity telling me how I can do this? Isn't that kind of being a chicken or wimpy? To really beat this I thing,* I thought, *at this early stage I need to write my own story or else it will be faked. I'm already getting into kind of a groove here and figuring some things out.*

There is an organization dedicated to this illness. It's called "No Stomach for Cancer." But everything on their site, at first glance at least, is depressing. Stories of death and sadness. So I stayed away from that for the time being.

Again, I would be wrong here as well. I was a victim of ignorance in the early stages, overly optimistic and confident with too many go-get-em, rah-rah influences. Everyone wanted to see me be strong, and so I was. And it was easy early on, before I was broken by surgery and incessant treatment.

I later found out I would need all of the stories, inspiration, information, hope, prayers, and help I could get from anywhere to figure this out, and most of all, to recover. I couldn't be picky or judgmental, claiming that someone's aromatherapy, acupuncture, diet, or guided healing imagery was too weird for me. I needed it all, and over the months I endured this, I slowly started to absorb every bit of help I could get my hands on.

I know what you're thinking by now. *Damn, this is going to be a depressing book*. Well, the thing about cancer is that it casts a pall over everything. It dulls the happiness of every situation, especially if you feel physically horrible, as I did for the first two years.

So I tried very hard to switch my perspective. Instead, what most would consider to be normal occurrences I thought of as tender moments, if for nothing else than because I was just happy to be alive to see them. But this is oh-so difficult to do. Because you stand on the sidelines of exciting home and work developments, you are relegated to attending only a portion of events, programs, parties, and spontaneous gatherings, you sit on the couch in pain when everyone is having fun or being productive. It gets better from here, I promise, and there is a happy ending somewhere in here. There's gotta be.

Mortality

Within the first week, my consciousness was heightened when it came to my mortality. A lot of people still didn't know what I was going through. But all of the random references that seep into everyday life regarding death were like a boldfaced, underlined, italicized cruel joke to me. Of course, there's the news on TV and in the papers, which is just riddled with instances of death. Things like house fires, car accidents, Darren Daulton's brain tumors—at least I'm not all of those people. I do prefer my situation to a sudden or imminent death, of course.

But then there was the more subtle stuff. I sat in a meeting, for instance, with a volunteer group at work, and a casual discussion surfaced about which is the better funeral home in town. The going rate is $600 for a two-hour viewing, I found out. I perked up with unusual interest during this conversation and instantly decided, *if I go, I'm definitely going with my favorite nearby funeral home instead of another rival one*. Better price, and I knew the owner pretty well. Plus, his facility was in an awesome historic home in town.

Other references abounded. There was the random talk of "getting hit by a bus" during work conversations. "Just in case I get hit by a bus," one would say, "I left the keys to the gate here."

Other clichés hit me hard too. One day I stared at the "What's On Your Bucket List" sign at the YMCA, which was posted in big cutout cutesy bubble letters. It looked harmless and fun to most, but very sinister to me. I almost ripped it off the wall. I really did.

"Screw the bucket list," as I said in between workout sets in my head, "for now I just want to survive."

Another day, just a few days after my diagnosis, I walked down the Ocean City, New Jersey, boardwalk past the rows of benches with memorial plaques that said things like "In loving memory of Ryan Calder, Husband, Son, May he Rest in Peace (1965-1997)." Realizing Ryan was only thirty-two when he died, I wondered how he passed away and if it was preventable.

A few weeks later, I attended my first funeral since the diagnosis. It was different for me to attend a funeral now. I couldn't help but think that this foreshadowed my own death.

Of course, it would be different in many ways. At this one, surrounded by lilies and about fifteen family members, Finn started to cry and Becky started to cry and I started to cry. Although none of us actually said it, we all knew that we cried about me and not my wife's ninety-eight-year-old grandmother in the casket at the front of us. It was about me. All of the talk about meeting Jesus and being with dead loved ones, the cheesy organ sound, the songs, the testimony—it all resonated because we knew that I could be up there in a casket pretty soon.

The fact was I didn't know where I would be buried if I did die or where my service would even be, which hurt even more. I was like a lost lamb. That was something I had to get figured out, and soon.

As I sat there in the chair, listening to the funerary remarks, I pondered what it would be like to die. Would it be like Bruce Willis in the *Sixth Sense,* wandering through the world, or like Patrick Swayze in *Ghost*? Would I float up into the sky? Or would it be nothing but blankness, darkness, and coldness?

I once read a book, *90 Minutes in Heaven*, about this guy in a horrific car crash. And he was left for dead but somehow miraculously came back to life. In the book he describes what he saw and felt in those ninety minutes "in heaven," and it's very hard to argue with this guy. I mean, he was dead, literally, and then came back to life. So he had to "go" somewhere. His brain had to shut down and his spirit went off to heaven. I really believe that. *I should read that book again now, since I have a different perspective. Instead of just being an inspiring story, it would now be field research for me.*

Leaving the funeral, I thought of other books that spoke to me more at this moment than ever before. What feels most relevant now to me is the book-turned-movie, *The Time Traveler's Wife*. It's a compelling story about a man who uncontrollably jumps through time. One moment he's with his wife, or family, or at work, and the next he's naked at a different point in his life, and he has no way to control this at all—kind of like a seizure. He finds out through his travels that he will die young, but he doesn't know exactly when. He falls madly in love with a woman; they marry; and he fathers a beautiful girl named Clare. He is powerless to know when, how, and where his death will happen. Even after he's technically dead, his former self appears to his daughter because when he was still alive in the past, he had time travelled into the future years beyond his own lifespan.

Will I die and do that to my kids? Will they think that they see me during a field trip to a museum in Philly even after I'm dead? Will they vividly dream about me like I dream about my dead father?

Other parallels come to mind. Perhaps I'm more like Alexander Supertramp from *Into the Wild* by Jon Krakauer, the man who checked out of life and wandered into the Alaskan wilderness. Or maybe I'm more like Henry Lightcap from *The Fool's Progress,* my favorite book by Edward Abbey, who is dying and travels back east to his childhood roots. These are protagonists with a slight anti-hero element from two excellent authors, and they die in the end, in solemn glory.

No matter where I was in these early stages, my mind wandered from death back to life. I could be at home, watching a swim meet, or in a work meeting, but I couldn't help but think about my own death. I ruminated over other bad things that could happen to me, and whether I'd choose them over stomach cancer. Here's a small list of things I *used* to think would be completely devastating, completely ruin my life, but now I'd gladly take them over this:

- Colostomy bag—I'd do it, no problem.
- Loss of a limb—no worries at all. This would not be an issue for me.
- Diabetes—I always thought this would totally suck, but now I know it would not at all. Just having to worry about what you eat, and not getting fat, and also checking your sugar levels from time to time. It would be a breeze compared to this.

- Blindness—at least I could still be a good dad, and a good lover. I do live in a walkable town and would get a cool dog to help out. I would ditch the useless dog I have now.

- Wheelchair bound—that's a tough one, very tough, but I could still be a dad, I could still love my wife, I could still work and produce. I would know that I would have a long life ahead of me.

Think John Hope Franklin!

For that matter, I'd rather have a bunch of different kinds of cancer than this. I'd take Colon Cancer, for instance, which killed my father at age 54 any day over this. The survival rate is more than double what I'm looking at. Lymphoma or prostate or breast cancer or something else would be way better too.

But here's where I draw the line: I would not want to be a stroke victim, vegetable, or be in the shell of a body. Put my brain in a jar and somehow allow me to listen and be heard and I'm okay. But if I can't communicate, forget it. And also, I could not endure M.S., Parkinson's, or early onset Alzheimer's. *Phew—now I really know where the line is and I'm learning a lot about myself.* The magic of cancer: forcing these issues to the surface!

During one of my early appointments, as we walked down a hallway at the hospital, I looked at the directional signs for different cancers. I realized in that moment another thing that I would not want to get. I would not want to have rectal cancer. I mean, seriously, how I could possibly sit around a table with my staff and announce that I have rectal cancer? Or imagine chatting at a cock-tail party and hearing, "I'm so sorry about Rob's penile cancer." Thank you, Lance, for making testicular cancer manly and discussable.

When the news did spread of my illness, it was a sur-prising phenomenon. I know it sounds like a cliché, but it spread like wildfire. When most people say that news spreads like wildfire, they probably mean that it spread like a crazy instant blaze, like the Santa Ana winds blowing flaming tumbleweeds mixed with brittle pine tree fire across the Sierra Nevada, scorching everything in its way. But when I say it in regards to the announcement of my cancer, I imagine a gentle fire that started one day and slowly spread and crept across the landscape. It might have hit a vein of dry grass in one spot and shot off or caught a wind one day and spread exponentially, but it was gradual.

Some people found out through formal means, such as an email sent, a meeting held, or a conversation on the phone. Others discovered this through second, third, or fourth parties. Some people still didn't know a month later. How do you announce to the world that your world has been turned upside down? Certainly not through social media, which saps the situation of its seriousness. Within a month, it seemed like the entire town of West Chester—my West Chester—knew.

During those first few weeks, when I fell asleep at night or for a nap, it was hard not to ignore the pain in the center of my chest. That I can actually feel this damn tumor is like the ultimate insult. It literally hurts me most of the time.

I imagine my cancer being like a throbbing chunk of kryptonite lodged into my body or like a black hole that sucks all of my energy, all of my happiness into it. The minute those positive things are generated—a laugh, a tender moment with my wife, an inspiring thought—the antimatter of that black hole immediately sucks them into nothingness and all that's left is the cancer, the glowing green kryptonite. That's why I want so desperately to get it out of my body.

All I know is this: I can make it through this, which I will do if I can. And when I do make it through, I tell myself, *Nothing will ever scare me ever again.* Nothing, never, ever.

Hopefully, that's what this is all about and the end of the story is me getting on with my life and all of my family being strong, close, bound together, all deeply in love with each other, sticking up for each other, shrugging off difficult times, letting the little things go. We will all be strong, and none of us will ever be scared ever again. Like most things I thought early on, this was easier thought than acted, as fear was alive and well through the entire process. Hopefully, there will be a day when that fear is gone.

"John Hope Franklin," I say to myself. "Just keep thinking of John Hope Franklin."

CHAPTER TWO
My "Body Love" and Family

Frederick Douglass endured a painful early life but was able to turn his life into a positive force that changed the world. The renowned abolitionist and civil rights activist was involved with the Underground Railroad and fight for civil rights. He also had strong ties to West Chester, Pennsylvania.

This chapter provides a background into my own life and ambitions and how they were cut short by this disease. It discusses my wife and kids, their reactions, and their roles in helping me fight this horrible disease.

THE last time I felt this kind of hopelessness was, crazily, just after 9/11. We got married on September 7, 2001, and it was a storybook "Ralph Lauren"-looking wedding. Or at least so we were told by our 150 guests.

The only hitch was, when I said my vows, I blanked on one part. Instead of saying "in abiding love" I said "and my body love." From the moment on, she was my one and only "body love," and we laughed every time we said it.

Our reception was at a Du Pont mansion in North Delaware. It was beautiful and unreal and sublime in all ways. After the reception, we stayed in room 1701, a corner room of the new Penn's Landing Hyatt in Philadelphia with a sweeping 180-degree view of the city. We took a few days off to gather our thoughts, dawdling around our house, which we rented from my mother.

Four days later, we boarded our plane bound for the U.S. Virgin Islands, ready for takeoff at 9 a.m. on Tuesday, September 11. My wife hated flying, and it was no different on this day. In fact, she needed an early morning vodka tonic to calm her nerves before we took off. What happened next didn't help. Immediately after boarding, we received a phone call from a close friend.

"Are you okay?" she asked.

"Yes, of course we're okay!" we replied. *How could we not be okay?* I thought to myself. *We are on a plane to paradise on a picture-perfect morning.*

"Well," she murmured, "there was a small plane that crashed into a building in New York." She considerately understated the truth, and we thought nothing of it.

Then there was a second phone call. This time, she spoke with more concern when she asked, "Are you guys still taking off?" She mentioned the second plane.

Then five minutes later the pilot announced that we must permanently de-board the plane. The stewardesses were crying, and I knew immediately that something was horribly wrong. I think we were the only ones who knew how serious this was.

As we left the plane, some insensitive jerk exclaimed, "I can't fucking believe this! This airline can never get anything right! They always fuck everything up!" He ranted as he ripped his bags from the overhead compartment and stomped off the plane. Little did he know, everything changed for everyone that day.

The National Guard swarmed the airport like we were in a developing country. Becky's father picked us up, and we spent the rest of the week watching television in utter shock with the rest of America. We waited a few days, wondering if the authorities would let planes fly again and if we would go on our honeymoon.

That was a hopeless feeling. And just like my cancer, nothing would ever be the same again. Just like 9/11, the day I found awoke from that endoscopy, July 22, 2013, was a sinisterly beautiful day. There was not a cloud in the sky, and it was ultra-bright and sunny. And just like 9/11, everything in my life would be judged by its proximity to that moment in time. Everything fell into two categories: events that occurred in the period of innocence before and those that occurred after.

I first met Becky almost exactly thirty years before my diagnosis. It was 1983, and we were awkwardly entering the sixth grade at a private school in suburban Philadelphia. She was Becky Gadsby then, spry and tomboyish, an athletic twelve-year-old.

I was goofy, clumsy, and infinitely unsure of myself. We joke about how, but for the first year, I actually thought her name was Ashley. Ashley was another girl in the class, and they looked nothing alike. How I got that idea in my head, I don't know. A sixth grade boy's mind is wondrous, strange, and horrid thing, actually. I was no different.

By the eighth grade, I had developed a full-blown, incurable crush. She was so beautiful and so confident. I remember the clothes she wore then just like it was today. The tightly-fitting cream-colored pants made me swoon. The peach-and-orange striped sleeveless sweater revealed enough to keep my imagination going. The smell of Calvin Klein's "Eternity" still makes me think of her today, because she wore it every day through the eighth grade.

"Lukens! Lukens!" the teacher would snap as I day-dreamed about Becky, appearing to nap. I used to sit there in class, thinking I was so clever to get a view of my goddess. I put my head on my desk and acted like I was sleeping. But instead of sleeping, I angled my 1985 Timex calculator watch to the perfect angle so I could stare at her undetected in the reflection. I would soak her reflection in to my heart's content.

Through high school we hung out with similar friends. The crush continued in full force and developed secret-ly as we finished high school. If I had only known how much pain she was in then, going through some serious stuff at home and in her personal life, I would have cared deeply for her then and there, but she seemed to have it all together.

My crush was so obvious that I remember my parents asking, "Rob, who's the prettiest girl in school?" I quickly blurted out "Becky Gadsby!" And that's the way it was. I would have dropped anything for her, done anything to have her as my girlfriend, and yet I shyly remained on the sidelines, watching her be the center of school attention.

After graduation, we became good friends. She would write to me in college, talking about her experiences in Michigan while I was trapped in a small, dry Pennsylvania town. We had separate girlfriends/boyfriends, but just being in contact with her was enough for me at that point.

I never dreamed that we'd actually be together sometime in the future. I fed off of the thought that we could even talk, write, and hang out alone together every now and then. I remember one magical time when we were home on spring break listening to music in my room. We were both going through that Bohemian stage of the early twenties, and it brought us a little closer.

When we both moved back home, we hung out a lot. We'd go drinking almost every night of the week at the bars until at least midnight, shooting pool, chugging beer, and watching late-night football games. There were late nights partying at peoples' homes or apartments, having a good time for the sake of it. I was a long-haired intellectual type, and she the short-haired artist. We were both beautiful physical specimens of twenty-something human beings.

Then, in fall 1997, it finally clicked. At a party with friends, the floodgates opened up. Over the next two months, I fell completely head over heels in love with her. It was all perfect, I thought, her and me finally, after fifteen years of playing games—we were together.

But the wheels quickly fell off the bus. She wasn't ready for me for various reasons. I was so angry and devastated. Like kryptonite in my stomach, sucking away my happiness, it sent me into a painful tailspin.

Months went by with minimal contact. And then it was my turn to inflict pain. When she was ready for me, I acted like I couldn't care less. Letters and phone messages went unanswered. This no-man's land dragged on for a year.

Meanwhile, I was dealing with some serious stuff of my own at home as my father was struggling with colon cancer in his early fifties. My dad died, and I was sent rudderless into the world.

I'm not sure when or why this painful behavior ended. I just remember a moment of clarity in 2000, realizing that perhaps the path to love and happiness is not a straight line, but a little more like a game of *Candyland* or *Chutes and Ladders*. You go forward a little bit, get stuck in the gingerbread stickiness or whatever else it is, shoot up a couple of levels, fall down two more, and then you find your way eventually to the top. I guess there's really no way in those games literally to get stuck forever. If you keep playing, the odds say that you will eventually make it to the top. And we did.

The end for me, the prize, was her. And my love for her was forged in special places. She went on vacation with us to Hilton Head Island, among my top three places on the planet. We kissed on the beach and shared drinks late at night when everyone else on the island seemed to be asleep.

I decided that I wanted to marry her in April 2001. I remember that vividly too. I was on a plane, talking to a total stranger as we both left a museum conference in St. Louis.

For some reason, I told this total stranger, "I'm going to go home and propose to my future wife." My seatmate seemed surprised but not shocked.

I arranged breakfast at a local café with her father. He knew what it was about and promptly gave his blessing over a breakfast of eggs, hams, hash browns, and hot coffee.

Then, a month later, I proposed to her on a windy, super-bright late afternoon on Memorial Day weekend 2001. Oddly enough, it was like our wedding day, 9/11, and the day I learned I had cancer. We were on Madaket Beach in Nantucket. The clouds were super-illuminated, and we were alone except for a woman walking her dog on the beach and a silent log that witnessed the event. I brought along a camera, but the batteries were dead.

While discussing something fairly mundane, I worked up the courage to turn towards her on my knees and present the ring and say, "I will love you forever, and I know it, and I would like you to marry me." She was shocked by this and said "Yes!" I tried to click the camera, but it didn't work. So the next year, for our anniversary, my artist wife painted the scene, and we have the painting hanging in our bedroom. It's better that way.

So that brings us back to 9/11, and that same sinking black hole feeling in my belly, except this one will take surgery to remove and just might kill me.

It's been almost twelve years since we got married, and I always thought that twelve years was a big deal. Why? Because of the big "D"—we've seen people get divorced around now. Disillusioned and taking everything for granted, marriages fall apart. I figured if we could make it twelve years without any major marital problems, we were good forever. I never thought that cancer and the specter of death would be the greatest threat to our young marriage.

Looking back now on all of the stupid fights, I cringe at how senseless they were. There was Mother's Day in 2013 when we barely spoke, or times when I selfishly freaked out because dinner was not ready for me when I came home after a long day. They've always stemmed from me not being sympathetic enough and being an idiot.

Our fights always went down like this: we would spend one whole day of silence, wearing each other down, a war of attrition. I was the most stubborn and rarely gave in. It was always her; she'd come to me crying, I'd say "I'm sorry," then we'd get on with our lives.

One year she decorated the whole damn Christmas tree by herself because we got into some dumb argument. There were conflicts, there were disagreements, but they were not fundamental. Now we are way beyond that kind of behavior. Since my diagnosis, we rarely have silly fights over stupid stuff because we do not want to waste a day not talking.

Now, I have to simultaneously survive, help her and the kids be happy with me as I continue being a dad and husband, and also prepare for my possible death. That brought me to life insurance. Why couldn't this happen when I was working at the U.S. Capitol a few years back? Back then, we used to joke "You'll end up with a half-million dollars if I," as Abbie would say when she was a bit younger, "got 'kicked in the bucket.'" Between that and Social Security, she'd be set.

I have to say, and it sounds counterintuitive, but some of the most content moments with my family came in the first six weeks since my diagnosis. There were tender moments of pure love. We lay extra-long in bed, enjoying big family hugs. Yesterday was our twelve-year anniversary, and I always told Becky that if we made it twelve years, we could make it forever.

Just to explain to the world and particularly my children, here is why I think that our marriage will last forever (or at least as long as I last): I married a woman who is incredibly attractive. First and foremost, you must love someone completely. But what seals the deal is she's downright sexy, and at forty-one, she's even more beautiful than ever. That was by design. You need to marry someone who you will always believe, truly believe, deep down in your heart, is smokin' hot. I did that.

Just as important, I married someone who is full of selfless love. You will know it when you see it. You will know it when that person does things for you that bring them no benefit. You will know it when they grab your hand and squeeze it tight for no particular reason. Becky is full of love: love for me, love for our kids, and love for our family. She is not perfect. Sometimes she's a bit clumsy, sometimes she does things that don't make sense to me, and sometimes I wish she'd be a little more proactive. But this is the yin and yang of love—she is she, and I am I, and we are perfect together.

Here's the other thing, especially for my kids when it comes to love: Don't worry about the money. Don't worry about who can support whom and what they can do. That will all fall into place. Gosh, I'm a historian married to an artist, and we are fine. Don't marry someone for money, ever. It's a stupid idea. Just get a better life insurance policy!

And don't let money ever factor into any family relations, close or extended. Don't ever get financially involved in a significant way with family—it will lead to disaster. If you loan family money, expect them not to pay it back and consider it a gift. If they pay it back, great. If not, then you need to decide in advance that you don't need it back and it won't affect your relationship.

Faith is important. You must both have the same spiritual values. This is something you cannot compromise on. You must both believe in God and be willing to pass those values on to your family. This is, admittedly, one of my weaknesses—being a spiritual leader of this family. I need to step up my game in that department, and I plan on starting today.

Becky is hot and only forty-one years old—quite a catch, actually. Would it be better to rip off the Band-Aid now and die and let her get on with things? A long, drawn-out death would drain her. *Every memory we make now will be tainted with the taste of imminent death. There will be nothing really, truly happy if this death sentence is certain.* We would all just be acting like we're happy to eke out a few more good memories.

At that moment, just before diagnosis, I had never been so content with my kids, my wife, my home, my town, my career, and my friends and family. They all blow my mind. I've been so blessed and hope I can enjoy them for a while longer.

At the beginning of my diagnosis, this was all the calm before the storm, and I really had no idea what lay ahead. I thought that I'd either live or die, but instead I spent the next two years in tortuous recovery, medically-induced side effects, pain, nausea, extreme weight loss, and ultimately horrendous psychological and physical pain.

Early on, when I tried to bring up the obvious notion of my death—"Becky, you do realize that there's a good chance I will die"—she seemed to shut down. My goal was to start a conversation and work out a contingency plan in case I didn't make it.

Even about six weeks in, we still didn't really talk about death. We avoided the 28 percent chance that I would live past five years, which I'd decided to bump up to 50 percent based on age and grit. We took care of my will and discussed the "what if" with a financial advisor, but I thought she didn't know about how high the chances were that I wouldn't make it.

Finally, I cornered her one night before bed, saying, "Listen, there's a very good chance I might die, and I need you to think about what you will do next without me." She still shut me out, and somehow the conversation transitioned to a jovial one.

She said then, "When we are both down, we can be happy in our misery together." We laughed at that. We were so ignorant early on about what we were up against, but I wouldn't trade that ignorance now for anything. Then we fell asleep in bed, praying, holding each other in complete and utter love and affection. We were simply soaking it in.

I said, "The days last forever, and I wish we could just speed all of this up and get it over with and get on with things."

To that, she replied, "I wish we could slow things down."

I abruptly sat up, facing away from her where she couldn't see the look of shock on my face. The implications of her retort were very clear to me; that she and the kids just want more time with me because I might not make it. We should "slow time down," like she said.

I paused for a minute to soak it in and quickly covered up the raw bare truth of the matter: that she was right. "Yes, you're right, we're having some special times right now despite all of this crap." But the awkwardness hung there in the air as I drifted to sleep, thinking "she knows how bad this is, but she just doesn't want to talk about it."

I almost talked about the 37-50 percent chances of my survival right then and there, along with my plan for her to learn new work skills for a post-Rob world. I had planned to line up meaningful, low-stress work for her with full benefits through my many business contacts. My plan was to make her self-sufficient.

In January, two months after my surgery, I tried to bring it up again. We had a very frank but brief conversation about it all. She hated it when I hinted at dying anytime soon, but it brought me comfort to confront that fact. To her, she would say, "It's terrifying and I can't go there!" *This "building a team and having a plan" thing is going to be a whole lot more difficult than I thought.*

Even eighteen months later, after my surgery, I awkwardly tried to introduce the topic again because I worried about her and the kids without me. We were on the couch, kids in bed, and I sprung it on her. Instead of the thoughtful, sympathetic reaction I expected, since it was my death we were talking about, she exploded in a hailstorm of tears and left the room.

"You threw too much at me at once," she said.

"But how can I even talk about this with you?" I replied. *Should I leave secret little notes?* I thought. "Just tell me, please—how can we talk about me dying and planning for it?" I pled. "We need to envision a future without me and figuring that out now might not be a bad idea, instead of when I'm choking my last few breaths on a respirator!"

I couldn't get out the rest, but what I would have said was "that we would live every day like it means something and, while building skills to live without me, she'd be building skills that are useful now with me." That was all I wanted to get across.

At the same time, of course, it immediately occurred to me that the best way to solve financial needs for Becky was for her to remarry, to find another me. And that was not really my dilemma; it was hers and for her to deal with. I couldn't possibly expect her to just stay a widowed spinster for the rest of her life. That would be so selfish of me.

But perhaps she could tell me now that I'm the only one and really believe that in her heart or fake it really well while I'm still on the planet. After all, I'm not going to be here to see what happens next anyway. And I think that she would really believe that to be the case now, even if she changed her mind later.

Other thoughts come across my mind as I ponder this unavoidable fact that I will probably be replaced. I've seen examples of widows remarrying and the marriage going awry, so I already assume that the next guy will be some jerk or not nearly as good to her and the kids as me. I should probably seek out examples of someone getting on with their life with a good person for a little bit of macabre inspiration for me. Like everything else in this situation, seeing real life examples are helpful for me in all areas.

Then my mind wandered to the absurd. "What if there was some kind of a special dating service for spouses with a terminal disease to arrange a marriage, or at least a few dates, ahead of time?" We could all get together as a group.

The only person I'd trust is a widower, not someone divorced or a bachelor who could never get it right. It would be nice if he was pretty rich, actually, which Becky deserves after putting up with me, the historian. And my kids could come along too. It would be a group date!

Then a worse thought crept in. What if someone I knew, perhaps an ex, or someone who had their eye on her the whole time, swooped in right after I died? They might appear during a moment of weakness for her. She might be alone and sobbing and vulnerable and looking for comfort. He might hold her and say he'll take care of her and she'll never have to worry about anything again.

I'm already starting to have dreams of her being with other men. Last night, I dreamt that there was a group of us at a party, and she just mentioned in casual conversation that she had been with so and so. And then later in the dream, she fell asleep surrounded by two other guys, all snuggled together. I know that she would never do any of this, but it's my mind telling me that I'm not enough of a husband now alive and weak, or dead.

Regardless of her remarrying or not, the irony doesn't escape me that the cancer trauma is naturally preparing

Becky to be alone without me. Ever since my surgery, she has basically been a single mom struggling to hold her life together because my abilities, physical and mental, are so limited. I can't take the kids out for fun activities; help with picking them up; and so on.

I'm worse than useless because I'm high maintenance too. She is learning to pull her resources, allow people to help her, and be strong for her kids, thinking positively and protecting and shielding them.

She even chaired an incredibly successful fundraising event the week after my surgery. In the heart of all of this, she got up in front of 300 people and gave a stellar speech. I was so proud of her even though I couldn't witness it—my Becky!

She's growing in incredible ways and impresses me every day, in every way. Even her driving in the city and navigating things on her own is impressive. She's even busier now with work than she's been in years, and somehow she's keeping it all together, being strong. I'm totally in love with her.

She goes to parties by herself. She takes the kids everywhere without me. She runs my work's fundraising meetings without me. She meets with people and conducts business in her job without my input. She is slowly coming not to need me anymore. In fact, I think she needs to escape from me from time to time to be in the normal world. It's fine, it's okay. Everything about me right now is completely tainted by cancer, and I know and understand that. I'm proud of her; she's growing stronger every day.

I hope that all of these unplanned training and experiences work. I believe that's the case; that this is building her into a new person. There was not anything wrong with her before, but she's stronger, more confident, and doesn't take crap from anyone. People love her and trust her. She's a total powerhouse, a total package of a forty-one-year-old, twenty-first-century woman.

A year after my diagnosis, when I'm still recovering from treatment and waiting for another scan, I see that she's really become the head of the household. She is the one who cares for the kids and makes decisions. Yes, I still technically bring home the bacon, but she handles everything else. We have become a matriarchal family. She's the one who handles all of the kids and me—all of our needs. She sets the rules, and I'm powerless. This is all good, all training for being a single mom.

Will it be the same for me? Will I become stronger if I make it? As I get deeper into this so-called recovery, I feel just the opposite. My strength is sapped and spirit is broken. I've certainly lost my mojo.

However, hopefully, somehow, someway, I will build up too and *use this to make me unstoppable*. Even more important, *I want to be a better father because of this*. I want to be there every second for my kids, which would be a 180-degree turn from where I am now.

The day before our twelfth anniversary, before my surgery, I realize that I have done absolutely nothing for her. I've purchased no gifts, no cards, and no flowers. So I rush out to the store. When I'm there, I feel like I'm going to explode. I'm not even man enough to give her a proper anniversary, and it's not even the cancer's fault. It's my own fault for allowing the cancer to distract me.

I walk through the soup aisle, and my anger grows to the point that tears are welling in my eyes, and people are looking at me. I want to take my hand and, like a snowplow, scrape off a whole row of Campbell's soup cans and send them catapulting onto the floor.

In the card aisle, I just put my hands in the air and yell "What's the point!" and I say it aloud, much to my own surprise.

The flower selection disappoints me. Nothing there actually smells like flowers, just plants, so I quietly but forcefully curse the inadequate Asian lilies and cheesy-looking colored carnations and stomp away.

In the ice cream section, I want to clear the shelves again and scream at the happy people who walk past me living their lives as if they have nothing to worry about. Self-pity, which I loathe, overcomes and overwhelms me. I have to leave. I grab my items quickly, pay, and scowl at everyone along the way. I am so angry.

Yesterday, nearly a year after my diagnosis, I had a complete meltdown. I could have had the same meltdown a year ago, but there's a secret in my belly now that only God knows the answer to. And the suspense is killing us.

After my meltdown, Becky said, "Perhaps tomorrow will be the end of the world, and we won't have to worry about any of this."

"I hope so..." I replied.

Kids

"Guys, come here for a minute. Mommy and Daddy have something important we need to tell you." That was how the *big* conversation began.

"You know how Daddy had a test the other day to see why he's having so much pain in his belly?" I asked. They nodded their heads.

"Well, Daddy has something in his belly that the doctors are going to have to remove," we told them. "It's serious, but Daddy's going to be okay."

We kept it light when we first told the kids because we did not want to overwhelm them. We said I was sick and not feeling well, so to please take it easy on me, and Mommy as well. They agreed. The "C" word, however, didn't come up, yet.

"Why is Mommy crying too?" my six year old son Finn asked. "Is she sick too?"

"No," we replied. "Mommy's crying because this all makes her sad."

A few days later, we took care of the inevitable. We had to tell them it was cancer and tell them soon, because what if they overheard a phone conversation or something?

"Remember when we told you about Daddy being sick the other day?" I told them. They nodded again. "Well, it's actually cancer, but the doctors are going to get it out, so I'll be okay."

I tried to put a positive spin on it. "Did you know that you will be special?"" we asked. "You will need to be strong," we continued, "but you will be one of a few kids *anywhere* around that has a parent with cancer." We realized later that this parent cancer card had limited playability in the real world.

"They even have a special overnight camp for kids like you, and it's totally free!" I exclaimed. "I don't think you'll be able to go this summer," I continued, "but maybe next!"

The kids saw right through this attempt to make them seem special.

When Finn heard the "C" word, he promptly said, with genuine concern "Are you going to die?!"

I immediately replied, "No, I will be fine."

This was *not* how the experts tell you to handle these things. There was an article I just read on the NPR website saying that you should not deny that death is a possibility in cancer situations. Instead, you should say something like, "Daddy's going to do the best to make sure that doesn't happen," or something else wishy-washy. My kids would have seen right through that too, so at this point, I thought it was best to ignore NPR's advice and flat-out deny it.

Finn followed by saying "But that's how Loden died!" Loden, our eight-year-old Vizsla, died a few years ago from cancer. He and my daughter Abbie remember me carrying him away alive and returning an hour later with him in a box, and then digging a ditch in the backyard. That was their only frame of reference when it came to cancer: Loden, and our four-year-old Golden Retriever, Digs, that died before they were both born. Digs' pictures were all over our house. So in their mind, cancer was a ruthless killer that inevitably ended with, as Abbie used to say when she was four, "getting kicked in the bucket."

Abbie then asked, "Is it going to take that long to get better?"

And I said "Yes, it's going to take a very long time."

When she found out later I was not drinking beer until I was declared cancer-free, she exclaimed, "No alcohol, Daddy? That's going to be very hard for you!"

Now I had something else to be concerned about: My daughter thought that the worst part of this treatment for me was my decision to not drink. Did I really drink that much before? Perhaps. I didn't keep this promise to myself, and, a couple of months later, I was helping myself to a beer or two at night just to get by.

It was so hard trying to tell them, trying to be positive but just aching and sobbing inside. It was awful seeing the confusion and sadness on their faces. It broke our hearts to have to tell them.

At the beginning, I told them it was like getting ready for a hurricane. I said, "This is like Hurricane Irene or Sandy," both of which we endured over the last two years. There would be lots of preparation, a lot of scary things, and then it would be really dark and gloomy and frightening for a while.

"Remember how the power went out and we couldn't watch TV and had to sleep in the basement?" I asked. They understood the comparison. "But then at the end the sun came out, and it all made for an interesting story, right?" They agreed again.

My children were six and nine when all of this started. They were, and are, happy children and beautiful. From the beginning, I was extremely concerned they would lose their childhood through all of this. So now that they knew, we tried to keep things as normal as possible in the beginning—at least when I could. We had soccer on Saturdays, Cub Scouts during the week, and I walked them to the bus stop when I could. I tried to help with homework and keep up physically.

The rest of the parenting thing seemed to be pretty straightforward. "Just be a dad," I told myself. "Make sure that they realize that I don't have the energy for piggy back rides up the steps to bed, or wrestling on the floor, or late sleepovers, or spontaneous soccer games in the alley—things like that."

Besides that, just be a good dad and try not to pull them down into a pit of sadness. And don't yell when you get angry at cancer, which is the hardest thing to do. It's so hard not to take this out on everyone.

But then, just like with Becky, my mind constantly and uncontrollably jumps forward to a time when I'm no longer here for them. I just can't help it. I don't mean to be negative, but it's the most natural reaction I can imagine. Trying not to think about it is like trying not to breathe for a while. It eventually creeps back in.

If I don't make it, I'll just be a blurred memory for Finn. Some fuzzy image of a happy dad, I hope, although that may change with my difficult recovery. I'm trying to remember when I was six years old, and it is hard. I remember sports, friends, moving to a new neighborhood, my school, my teacher, the playground, my brother, my family, and going to my grandparents in the country for fun.

When Digs died at age 4, we replaced her the next day with Loden. And when Loden died, we replaced him with our half-blind dog Hudson two weeks later. Will they replace me in a couple of months? Am I replaceable? Will I just be a fuzzy memory?

So instead of fighting it, I think it might be a good idea to share some of my limited wisdom about what I've figured out in the last forty-two years. Just in case I don't make it. I might not have the time to do this in person or at the exact appropriate time, so here goes.

There are some character attributes that they need to know about. Credibility, for instance, is key to long-term success. It is closely linked to likeability and reputation. There are so many corollaries to the credibility factor. You should not complain unless you absolutely must or else it will damage your credibility, and people won't believe you, follow you, or even listen to you when you have something valid to say. Do what you say you are going to do, be careful what you commit to, and don't overcommit or you will damage your credibility when you can't deliver on your promises. The reward is not in the saying but in the doing. The reward is when you cumulatively build up enough credibility that people associate that characteristic with you all of the time. Build your credibility, and people will respect you, and you will be successful.

The second thing is grit and resolve. Grit means trying again and again to achieve something you want and need and is good for you. Resolve means never giving up, unless it would be ridiculous not to do so or your dreams have changed.

The next is resilience. I will need a lot of this for the rest of my life, I suppose, and you will need it too.

Finally, believe in your dreams and they will come true. It's all about working hard and not expecting everything to happen immediately. It takes time to become good at stuff. Like your credibility, people want to believe you, so always tell the truth and don't overcommit to things or brag. Everyone, when you're young and old, will respect you for that.

My father always told me, "Lukenses never quit!" I took that to heart, but I knew that sometimes it's okay to quit, and those are the same times when grit won't help you. It's okay to quit when things are not working for you anymore, no matter how hard you try, and your dreams have changed.

If you do quit, though, do so gracefully and in ways that strengthen rather than weaken your relationships with those you might be leaving in some way. But do know that quitting should be a rare thing in your life—a last resort, or a way to get you to something better, like a job or school.

And then there are some specific things that I need to tell my children. For Abbie, just know that I love you and will always love you even if I'm gone. I will always be there for you providing inspiration, love, and a place to go when you are sad.

Abbie, keep that sparkle in your eye and turn my death into something positive. I know that you can. Continue to be bold, fearless, and do whatever you want to in pursuit of justice and what's right. Don't think that the first boy you'll fall in love with will be your husband—that's rare, but it's okay to fall in love anyway. Be careful with that, and listen very closely to what Mommy says when you fall in love.

When you get older, don't ever get into a car when your gut is telling you it's not safe. Call Mommy and she will pick you up, no questions asked.

Abbie, one of the most valuable lessons came from in a moment of clarity on July 7, 2014, just before my diagnosis. During a swim meet, I looked down on you from this grassy stage of about 300 kid swimmers. They had no idea that this was the stage for one of the proudest moments of my life.

My daughter was absolutely petrified to try the breaststroke. She had never been able to finish it in practice and pled with the coach that she couldn't do it. She cried and cried and said she hated swimming and would never do it again.

Instead of fleeing, she fought. She stuck with the team and nervously lined up on the starting block. She tried so hard, but off the block she was already dead last. But she kept going and going until, after all of the other kids were done, she finished to a friendly but raucous cheer. I have never been so proud.

As I told her, she faced her fear, persisted, and never gave up. Sometimes in life she'll be last, but other times she'll be first. She summed up any advice I could give her through her own actions.

When Abbie was born, she was breeched, so her head was not down towards my wife's pelvis, as it should have been, and instead she was upright in the womb, nice and comfortable. So she was born through C-section.

An interesting byproduct is that her right ear stuck out further than the other one for several weeks. Inside the womb her ear was folded over, creating this curious effect. Because of this, or maybe not, but at least coincidentally, she has always had an affinity for elves. When she was just days old, around Christmas, we watched a bootlegged version of the movie *Elf* about ten times over the course of a week while Becky convalesced. Maybe that seeped into her brain through her blurry newborn vision. I just don't know.

Her assumed elf-hood gave her magical powers. When she was young, she thought that she made everyday things happen, like phones ringing or weather patterns. She also believed that she could talk to our dog, Loden. She loved and still loves leprechauns and pots of gold and rainbows. We've looked for them before and built leprechaun traps every year in early to mid-March. And of course, her Christmas Elf, Jolly, is a treasure to her. Because of this, I believe that Abbie has a gift of happiness and loves people, just like a mischievous little elf would.

Your voice, Abbie, is that of an angel. Keep singing.

Again, assuming I won't be here to say these things at key points, I have some advice for my fair-haired son Finn. I love you more than you'll ever know bud, and that will stay with you forever. I hope I was a good dad. Know that I'm still with you every second of every day, hovering over you. Especially in tough times, look to me for guidance and comfort from the sky.

You are tough and gritty and that will get you very far in life. Know that you'll have to work well with people too—it's not just about hard work. You already do a great job at all of that. You will also need to persevere to accomplish all of your lofty goals.

When it comes to courtship, son, love is not a continuous, rising, shooting star but can come in different forms. Your mom and I dated but then broke up for a while before we completely fell totally head-over-heels in love. That may happen to you too, and don't be discouraged if love doesn't unfold perfectly for you. Love is not perfect—it's just love. My love for your mother is eternal.

Remember how smart you are and how quickly you pick up on new things. Don't be afraid of new things, and jump into new opportunities head-first. You are gifted in many ways.

Whereas Abbie was born with elf-like qualities, I have a theory about Finn's infancy too. When he was born, I swear we didn't swaddle him enough and because of that, he's been a bit wild ever since. We should have swaddled him tight so his arms couldn't flail. Because he could flail about and flip around, as my theory goes, it created a hunger for constant movement and activity. So he just always wants to go, he's intense and excels when he has a clear task right in front of him. Like swimming a race.

There was still one more thing, a secret that I needed to tell the kids. After my surgery, it took me nine months to tell them that I didn't have a stomach anymore. We withheld this information because we thought it would freak them out and they didn't need to know. However, the longer I went with my illness, the more often this came up in conversation with other people, and I feared they would overhear.

Abbie took it like a champ, or at least acted like it, jokingly saying, "They had to remove your stomach, Daddy, because you have such a big heart!" Finn didn't take it so well. He broke down crying, and then later Abbie did the same too. That's their differing styles. All of this happened on August 5, 2014.

Early on, I thought that the kids were the easiest and hardest part of my plan. I worried about them most in the post-Dad era that might be coming. However, as far as the "now" part, it was clear that I just needed to be a good dad. That would prove later to be much easier said than done. Being a good dad is hard when you're stripped of the manly prowess that allows you to play the role.

I find myself observing them very closely now. Before my surgery, when I was still feeling pretty good, I savored September evenings during soccer practice, with the sun slowly setting. I soaked in the view and smells and sounds. I heard my daughter giggling with her teammates and watched my son scurrying about the playground with friends he made five minutes before.

I closed my eyes and allowed it all to absorb into my body's every pore. My eyes are like lenses and my brain a video recorder to document every detail. Whether I live or not, these moments, I determined, must be burned into my brain. These silly, seemingly mundane instances with my kids take on extraordinary meaning for me.

Perhaps that's one of the lessons of this chaotic situation. If I live, these moments are to be memorized, committed to memory, and never forgotten or dismissed as unimportant. These moments are abundant. I read with my daughter at night, our heads gently touching at the top of her bed and our ankles intertwined at the bottom. I have conversations with Finn about Lego design as I drive him to the YMCA on a rainy spring Saturday. When Becky and I lie in bed, praying, the skin of our bodies deliberately has as many contact points as possible. Our hands, our arms, our heads, our torsos, and our legs and feet have all connected.

I find myself, when I've hit the one-year mark, withdrawing a bit from my fatherly role, as I feel like a failure or fake when I try to be a good dad. I know I shouldn't do this, but I do it anyway, spending more time lying down and listening to music, squirrelling away somewhere in our 2,200-square-foot home.

The irony hits me that it was the same with my dad. I knew that I needed to be there for my father when he was sick, and although I didn't realize how serious it was for him until nearly the day he died, I was an ass and wasn't there like I should have been. Am I doing the same thing now with my kids and wife by withdrawing in self-sympathy and selfishly savoring alone time when they need me most?

I, being a typical dad, sometimes explode at them. I send them to their rooms. I want them to just be quiet sometimes. I want their little health issues to go away, and I want them to be perfect human specimens.

My Dad

My most treasured possession is my father's college ring—a big hunk of gold with a large garnet stone in the center. I never wear it for fear that I'll lose it or it will be stolen. But

I know exactly where it is, and I wear it on very special occasions, like a talisman when I need extra strength.

My father went to La Salle University, and he was the first in his family to graduate from college. He worked his way through school, putting time in at a hoagie shop and at ushering at Franklin Field during the Eagles games. It doesn't get any more Philly than that—a Catholic schoolboy going on to college and serving up those hoagies.

Back to the ring. I learned that his parents were of a pretty stoic sort. I didn't know them that well, but my limited experience with them and stories I'd heard conveyed this to me. So as my father explained it, it was a big deal when they bought him an expensive class of 1969 La Salle College ring. He cherished this ring and wore it every day into adulthood.

One day, in about 1984 or so, he was dropping me off at soccer practice and opened his car door and the ring mysteriously flew off his finger. He was devastated and looked everywhere but couldn't find it.

Miraculously, in about 1997, he was contacted by La Salle. Someone, a treasure hunter with a metal detector, found it and called the school because of his inscribed initials and graduating year. In fact, they ended up on the front page of some kind of metal detector magazine. All of this, in my mind, added to the mystique of the ring.

My father, William Francis Lukens, was diagnosed with colon cancer at age 50 in 1996. He put up a huge fight and his attitude was remarkable, while he endured surgeries and chemotherapy. My mother was by his side as his nurse and advocate through it all. Unfortunately, it had spread to his liver. I had no idea how serious the metastasis to his liver made this until much later. I assumed that we would pull through, but he didn't. He made it almost four years, dying on February 20, 1999 at age 54.

When my father died, I was twenty-six, and I was in denial. I really hadn't thought it would happen. I was helping to take care of him but not really doing as much as I should have. I remember when he only had about six weeks left, which of course I didn't realize. He needed me home, and I wanted to go out with friends.

I selfishly whined and moaned, "What about me! Why can't I go out!" I yelled, "It's like I'm trapped here!" I was a stupid, self-centered twenty-six-year-old. It hurts me now to recall that moment. I want to go back and punch that twenty-six-year-old in the face.

I still remember watching him die. He was helpless in our dining room, which had been converted to a hospice ward. We removed the tables and chairs, and I had to tie the chandelier up to the ceiling in the middle of the room so that we wouldn't hit our heads when we went close to him.

On the day he died, he developed the death rattle—a sound I'll never forget. We knew it wasn't long. All of a sudden, it looked like he was choking. We told him how much everyone loved him, over and over. I kept saying my brother's name, Wil, who was 600 miles away and on his way to see him. Then he took his last breath. He was gone.

Now I think, *Will it be the same for me? Are we just waiting until the cancer aggressively takes everything over, until it infiltrates some vital organ, and I just start gurgling and die in a converted dining room?*

I dream about him often, still. My favorite is the dream when we are walking up a shallow stream, looking at beautiful rocks, walking towards the sun with everything glittering.

Other dreams of my father come pouring into my brain while I'm in the haze of chemo. In one chemo/drug-induced nap, I went deep into the recesses of my mind and there I found myself on a soccer team. We were playing soccer in the front yards of the neighborhood, and I was sorry that I couldn't help because I was sick. I walked into my house and saw my father in the kitchen, wearing his maroon shirt that he always wore, with the name "Maui" scribbled in yellow cursive midway down.

In this dream, I looked at him and melted into his arms and just said, "I'm sorry," and started sobbing. He didn't say anything back—he never does in dreams—but just looked at me like he meant to say, "I know, Rob, I know."

I was sorry for being sick and putting everyone through this. I was sorry for being a jerk when he was sick and not being more understanding. I was sorry that he never met my kids. I was sorry that I never appreciated him as much as I should have. And now, I watch my kids loving me and nurturing me and acting like I should have when I was watching my own father die.

Nearly two years later, I still wondered if it was better for me to die quickly for the sake of my family. Was it selfish to try to seek out a few more years while I gradually wither away? It might be better for everyone to rip off the Band-Aid and die quickly while they're all young. Becky could get on with her life, the kids will remember less, and the sadness won't hurt as much, perhaps.

I'm conflicted. Most days I just want them to have their dad a year, three years, five years, twenty-two years from now, like I did. I want them to have a dad when they have their first date, graduate from high school, and go to college. I want them to have a dad when they get married, when they're getting their first mortgage, having a baby, and need work advice. I want them to have a dad. And selfishly, I want that dad to be me.

CHAPTER THREE
My Work—On History and Cancer

John Hope Franklin, a preeminent African American historian, is one of the most famous historians of all time. He shrugged off stomach cancer at age seventy-one and lived into his 90s.

This chapter will focus on my career and how it intertwined with my life. Running an organization and fulfilling organizational dreams while battling cancer is not easy. This uplifting chapter will talk about how the people of my organization, the small museum, library, and the Chester County Historical Society, rallied around me and took the organization to new heights in my absence.

THAT first night when I learned I most likely had this horrid disease, that fateful July 22, 2013, my phone rang as I drifted asleep. I was almost asleep, wondering, in a Vicodin-induced sleep, what the hell to do next, when my phone buzzed—the alarm at my museum had been tripped.

"Hello, this is Central Station calling for Robert Lukens," the monitoring company relayed. "We have a report of an alarm in section 102 of the Chester County Historical Society," she informed me.

"Okay, I'll check it out," I replied.

As museum director and first on the dreaded "alarm list," it was my duty to rush to the facility and see what was going on. Most likely it was a false alarm.

As I wandered through the darkened museum in the middle of the night, I had a twisted thought. *How could I use this illness to advance my institution? Hey, it's me that we're talking about, so I should feel free to exploit myself, right?*

I thought of the funders lining up to help once they realized that a cancer patient was struggling to make this institution work. Bald from chemotherapy, I imagined sitting down with potential donors acting as if everything was normal. There was no way that they could resist, right?

Then again, it could backfire, and the opposite could happen. They might sense institutional weakness because of uncertainty. Like a Fortune 500 company, my institution's stock would plummet due to leadership concerns, and I would become a liability. The staff, Board, and community would resent me for dragging the organization down as a matter of vanity. People would uncomfortably watch me, wanting to tell me that I was actually harming things but not wanting to be the jerk that tells a cancer patient that they need to step down and abandon their passion. I could be like Chairman Mao or one of those other dictators. They would keep me stuffed and show old footage of me being alive just so people wouldn't freak out and go into a panic that crippled the nation.

When it came to work, what really angered me was that things were finally looking up after a dismal first two years of employment at my museum. This was my dream job, returning to the institution that gave me my start twenty years ago as an intern, to now run the place. I had a deep passion for everything about it—the collections, the educational programs, and most of all, the people who surrounded it.

Ironically, the morning of my first endoscopy, we had just gotten notice of a $300,000 bequest, which was a huge chunk of money for us. But the organization had always seemed snake bitten. In fact, they've had three staff die in the last ten years, including one at the helm. That was out of a sum total of only twenty staff!

So I was letting them down by perpetuating that tradition of bad luck because of bad health.

Up until that point, I thought that my life and my work situation were perfect. But being naturally skeptical, I knew that it all had to unravel somehow. Imagine this—I'm forty years old. I have two beautiful children, Finn and Abbie. I have a beautiful wife, who is an amazing wife and mother, and a kickass cook too. I run a museum in a historic town, the "Perfect Town," as West Chester touts itself. I live .8 miles from work and can walk there in less than fifteen minutes past outdoor cafés and shops.

It's a place filled with weekend festivals and friends. The kids play in the back alley for fun, a throwback to cities a hundred years ago, when kids played outside. We live in a historic 1928 craftsman-style home with original molding, a cute postage stamp backyard, with our nice neighbors packed in tight on all sides. It was ideal, and something, as my skeptical self thought, had to go wrong.

The museum had just gone through a hard time, and we remarkably were pulling out of it. I had started at this institution as a long-haired college kid in 1993 as a volunteer, looking to boost my grad school applications. Determined to become an academic historian but lacking in real book smarts, I overcame my late teenage stupidity through my genetic grittiness. This got me through grad school, but I continued to work at museums and historical libraries for additional income and career-related work experience.

Eventually I grew to love museums more than academic history itself. So in 1998, I ditched the idea of becoming a historian in the ivory tower and began working at my current museum, the Chester County Historical Society (CCHS) in West Chester, as Collections Manager. I was enamored, and that love of my profession continues today with incredible intensity. I spent my first summer internship at CCHS completely alone for three months in a windowless attic, cataloging teacups and padlocks, and fell in love with artifacts, teaching through tactile learning, and inspiring through the stuff of the past.

When I arrived back at the museum two years ago in 2011 as president, things were in shambles. The roof leaked into my office, so I literally had to use an umbrella if I wanted to work on my computer. Mold and window leaks pervaded the other offices. The iconic CCHS van, which I picked up brand new in 1999, was decrepit, covered with dents, and with doors literally about to fall off. The 242 sprinkler heads had been recalled, so the entire building and collection were in jeopardy of a false trip or malfunction. The elevator kept you guessing if you would make it out alive or require an emergency rescue. The aging HVAC system—our lifeblood for our sensitive treasures like letters by George Washington, Frederick Douglass's daguerreotype, and rare furniture—was on its last leg. The entire front terrace looked like it would collapse into the street. The cash deficit was 20 percent of our 1.2 million dollar budget.

Gradually, one by one, through sheer resolve, the staff and board worked through these things and connected to the community for help. By summer 2013, we were beginning to hit on all cylinders and putting things into high gear. There was an excitement in our halls. There was a buzz on the street. We were confident and strong.

When I thought about this, my perfect life, perfect town, perfect family, and this burgeoning success story that I was living in, I just knew that something had to go wrong. I knew this in the back of my brain and was constantly assessing the threats. Having the museum fall apart and losing my job seemed like the most likely possible source of any distress.

So, if you had to ask me before all of this cancer stuff what the weakest link was in our picture perfect life, it would be my job and its insecurity. That kept me up at night, not life altering diseases. I had a huge lack of mobility. I couldn't move us for another job like this anywhere. And I admittedly jumped around a lot in my previous positions, which would make me damaged goods and hardly employable. I had left a very secure cushy government job at the U.S. Capitol, where I was well paid and taken care of, for this current position. It was a huge risk to take on this one position that was the only job that could sustain this perfect life, perfect family, living in the perfect town.

So it was work that posed the greatest threat, the greatest possibility of this wonderful life crumbling down around me. It never occurred to me that cancer could take us down. Cancer? Bringing down my perfect life? The thought was as ludicrous as anything else I could imagine. Cancer, thus, blindsided me.

Once we discovered my illness, inevitably, work and life commingled even more than usual.

Early on, just after I discovered my fate, I found myself doing things like pacing around my office spontaneously chanting, "I will never take anything for granted ever again. I will never take anything for granted ever again. I will never take anything for granted ever again," over and over and over again. The staff didn't know yet. That day, I was awaiting lab results; one of many long days at the beginning when we were trying to figure out how serious this was.

As it slowly sunk in, I started thinking about the concrete good that could come out of this, like I did that night the alarm went off. *How about this for a fundraising tactic: If I get through this alive, I can say at the end that I'm a cancer survivor, and I could honestly say that I think donor money is better directed to my museum than a cancer cause. I can be a living example of someone who can have the credibility to say, "Give your money here." Why? Cancer money will be there from a variety of sources. But who will ensure that my and your legacy endure, the legacy of our times, for future generations? Only my museum. And only my museum looks after everything when we are long dead.* That would be my tactic.

When it came time to tell the staff, I tried to be very professional. I called everyone together for a special staff meeting.

"I have some very bad news to share with everyone," I said, trying to look very strong. "I've just been diagnosed with stomach cancer." Gasps and jaw-dropping occurred around the table. Tears almost welled up in my eyes, something I promised myself I would not do. *Don't show weakness, Rob,* I thought again and again in my head.

"However, I'm confident that I will be fine after surgery and treatment, and that this organization will be just fine," I continued. "I'm going to need to rely on everyone more while I'm out, but I know that everyone's up to the task."

We had an amazing staff. I told everyone I should be back in shape by Christmas, and I was so wrong.

Since I was in charge, my first instinct at work was to put things on lockdown, clear my calendar, shut everyone out, and keep the door closed. But then, the more I thought about it and talked to people, that was the exact opposite of what I needed. I didn't want to appear weak, for my family, my staff, my friends, and potential supporters. Shutting myself down and putting a "back in nine months" sign in the storefront would do just that. Second, I needed it to keep myself feeling useful, productive. Finally, for pure distraction, I needed to contribute so I could forget for a few minutes, or hours, about my affliction.

My own career plan from the beginning was very clear to me, although now it's all up in the air. I was to work at this museum for ten years, building the place up from nothing, really rolling up my sleeves and making this place work. And we were starting to get there, two years later. Very good things were happening after a chaotic first year.

Next step here at CCHS was to make this place shine. We would work with everyone to make it world class. And then, I said, I would retire from consulting. I would teach at a university for the tuition remission, as the kids were getting ready for college. And then I would just live out my life becoming wiser, richer, and more fulfilled as the grandkids came. We could live wherever we wanted—the Eastern Shore, New England, right here in West Chester—and do whatever we wanted.

That plan was shattered now. Now, I just needed to live. I wanted to live another five years, or hopefully ten, but preferably John Hope Franklin's twenty-two years! Now, I'm focused on accumulating wealth to protect this family, and do so as if on steroids.

The other thing I now needed to focus on was building my reputation quickly, because within five to eight years, if I'm alive then, I wanted to work for a big place with gobs of life insurance. My life insurance, as miniscule as it is, expires in nine years.

Being a leader and a cancer patient is difficult. Only two weeks into this, it really started cramping my style. I had to tell people about cancer and not cry. This is not easy, because every time I mention it, I see flashes of my kids, fatherless, advancing like a hyper-speed viewfinder in front of my eyes.

I pride myself on self-awareness, but every time I now meet with someone and need to be in an authoritative position, pitching my organization feels so forced because I'm so distracted. It's like that forced smile that one has to hold during the family picture when your rival brother is pinching you from behind.

Unfortunately, I have to fight my new default demeanor, which is a look of misery and tiredness on my face. It's in my body language too. I want to slouch and put my head in my hands. So I have to be incredibly conscious of it, or else I slide into this mode, which I'm sure is off-putting.

In the middle of a meeting, my mind wanders off in an instant to the next few months, the next appointment, my survival rate, and my real chances of making it while someone is talking about something that sounds so mundane to me now. How could it not? *I could die, dammit!*

Well, nine months later, what really happened with CCHS was incredible. More donations came in. My wife chaired the fall fundraiser while I was recovering for twelve days after major surgery, gave that heartfelt speech, and shattered fundraising records. The winter was brutal, but we survived and thrived. We instituted new consulting services and received unexpected donations, and even the HVAC system was replaced. Nearly 1.5 million dollars was raised for capital repairs, and I was chomping at the bit to come back to work and make all of our dreams for this special place a reality. I just needed this body to cooperate, and that question is still out there—am I well, now, almost a year later? No.

CHAPTER FOUR:
The Process—Surgery, Treatment, and Hell

G. Raymond Rettew, the pioneer of penicillin, was born and raised in my hometown of West Chester. He developed a way to mass produce penicillin from mushrooms and enlisted the whole town to do it. By 1943, he teamed up with the pharmaceutical Wyeth brothers to produce most or all of the Allied Forces' supply of the antibiotic, which changed the course of the war.

This chapter is meant not only to provide all of the details of what I went through and endured but also to show how such a process strips people of their humanity and, in particular, men of their masculinity in all ways.

"IT'S all about the bees under the ground."

Becky and I thought that was the strangest phrase we had ever heard. Was that some kind of new coping mantra among the cancer world that we had never heard before?

The woman who uttered these words sat across from us on a bench in the chemo waiting area. We had tried to make our own secluded little bubble, but this very well-dressed woman, in her sixties, infiltrated it and started mumbling about bees in the ground.

When she sat down across from us she asked, "Do you get cell phone reception here?" We were there on our first visit, so although we had good coverage then, it wasn't a trend we could attest to. All we could think was, *How dare she involve herself in our own little world of shock and denial?*

She looked up at us and said, "Well, I better continue on. It's all about the bees under the ground, you know." We sat there still thinking this must be some fancy lingo in the cancer world, all of which was so new and foreign to us.

After a few minutes, she dialed a number on her cell phone and starting talking. "Hi, I called the other day. Yes, I talked to so and so. Yes, do you think he could come out today and take care of the bees?" She continued on, "Yes, the bees. We are having a party tonight, and my grandchildren will be there, and I don't want them to play and walk along and have them all the sudden come out of nowhere and get stung when they least expect it." She rambled, "Yes, because the bees are living in the ground."

Oh, we thought, *she really was talking about the bees that had made nests and holes in her yard, underground!* It wasn't some crazy oath or saying that we had to learn now that we were in this inner sanctum called "cancer treatment." These were actual bees in the ground that attacked when you least expected it.

When Becky and I talked about it later, I learned her take on the "bees" and how appropriate those comments were for our situation. There you are, minding your own happy little business, your happy wonderful life, when you go walking through your yard, admiring your lawn and flowers that you've cultivated all season long, when *bam*, out of nowhere the bees under the ground attack. They come out of out of nowhere like cancer, stinging and biting you when you least expect it. "How awful is that? How terrible and unsuspecting. How unfair," she told me.

We wished with all our hearts that ours had just stayed the hell right where they were: underground, never to be seen. Now they filled every minute of this new, unwanted, stinging reality.

This was only a few weeks after we found out about my cancer, and we were already swept up in a whirlwind of confusing activity. There were scans, visits with oncologists, and the big decision of which hospital to go with, which all seems so rushed in retrospect. That was a decision that we think was right, but we'll never really know for sure. Co-pays and medical bills started rolling in.

When we first sat down with our oncologist and RN, it was as if I had arrived at a freshman orientation for cancer patients. They walked me through the side effects of the chemo, like extra sensitivity to cold, nausea, etc., and wrote out several prescriptions to deal with it. Then they handed me a kit, brightly colored, and sponsored by one of the pharmaceutical companies. It contained some materials, a nice bottle of lotion —"Because chemotherapy also makes your skin dry"—and a pill dispenser. *How nice and thoughtful,* I thought. I didn't realize we were getting freebies during my visit.

The doctors immediately scheduled me for surgery on August 19th to have my stomach removed and other organs, if need be. "This is an aggressive, serious mass, and it needs to come out as soon as possible," they said. When I asked how long the cancer had been there, the answer was "months to years." That it could possibly develop and grow so quickly in my body baffled me. And they were literally lining up an entire team of surgeons available to work on me the day of my surgery.

They said, "Plan on being out of commission for two months." Imagine that. I went from going about my daily business on July 21, to the diagnosis later that week, to the thought of having my stomach entirely removed forever, all within less than four weeks. So we had to get our lives in order!

And we did just that. I canceled appointments at work and cleared my schedule. Memos were sent around about dos and don'ts. I assigned an acting director to take my place while I was out. We lined up meals and people to help with the kids.

Then, at the eleventh hour, just days before the surgery was scheduled, I received an evening cell phone call from one of the surgeons. "Mr. Lukens, this is Dr. So and So," he relayed. "We have all discussed your case and decided that you should follow a different program, by having chemotherapy first, then surgery," he continued. "Results with this kind of cancer have been more successful when following this program," he concluded.

This method, they claimed, would hopefully shrink the tumor to make it more contained and catch any floaters that might have wandered undetected to other parts of my body. I would have surgery in about three to four months.

I still had surgery on August 19th, but they just put a port in my shoulder and poked around a bit with cameras in my belly to take a look through some routine laparoscopy. All looked relatively "good," with the cancer contained to my stomach.

Just four days later, with my wound still fresh from Monday's surgery, they started my treatment of Oxaliplatin, Epirubicin, and Xeloda.

They said, "We are hitting you hard with the toughest stuff available, and you will definitely lose your hair."

And it did hit me hard. I was tired, sick, and my whole body felt like it was pumped full of jet fuel. Other drugs, like steroids and antiemetics, helped, but also made me groggy, hyper, irritable, and overall not myself. I peed a rose color after each treatment. My body seemed like it was surreally detached from me.

There were some humorous moments too. While we were going through all of this, we became addicted to the wildly popular TV series *Breaking Bad*. Sometimes during chemo we would sit in our private suite, watching episodes of the series on Netflix. Just imagine: I was watching Walter White receive his chemo for entertainment, while receiving mine for survival. Becky and I chuckled when the nurses left the room, thinking they must have thought we were nuts for subjecting ourselves to such material. Eventually, the show was too much for us—too close to our situation in some ways—and we had to stop watching entirely.

I kept working through this. I couldn't work on treatment days, but I worked full-force on other days. I struggled to keep it all together and lead an organization while going through this intense regimen. I should have stopped, but a mixture of ignorance and sheer determination kept me going. I was on the radio and in videos. I made public speeches, kept long-range plans moving, and took care of the day-to-day needs.

After three treatments of this poisonous cocktail, the doctors scanned me, seemingly shrugged off the results as minor improvements, and then lined me up for surgery. *What were the last three months of treatment for?* I thought. Perhaps it didn't have the results they were looking for, but very little was made of them. Instead, it was full-steam ahead, scheduling to have my stomach removed.

I spent the next few weeks enjoying my stomach, eating out, visiting brewpubs to get the best beer, and generally doing whatever I could to live it up, knowing that I would never be the same again. We had professional photographs taken of our family, because I would be forever changed.

To make things even more interesting, I woke up one morning prior to the surgery with my arm swollen and throbbing with pain up to my neck. Four hours later, I learned I had two blood clots in my shoulder due to my port. By the end of the day, the doctor put me on a new regimen—daily shots of a blood thinner, Lovenox, injected in my belly indefinitely. The thought of giving myself a shot in the belly every day freaked me out. But I got used to it, like everything else, eventually.

I was so scared of the surgery. There was a chance that they would open me up, decide it was too far gone, and then stitch up my belly, telling my family there was nothing they could do. More likely, I would wake up a different human specimen.

I devised a coping mechanism for this anxiety and un-certainty and practiced before the big day. I imagined that

I was the baby Moses in Exodus. I would voluntarily place myself in this basket, in the hands of others, and trust that I would arrive well at the other side. When I arrived at the hospital that morning, I imagined I would be like a swaddled baby, placed in a basket and sent down the river like baby Moses. I would, like him, be entirely at the mercy of God.

I entered the OR waiting room about 7:40 a.m. on November 11, 2014, and arose from consciousness at about 9 p.m.

I was screaming, "My neck, my neck is killing me!" That's the first thing I remember about waking up from a seven-hour surgery. When I slowly came to, I looked down at tubes, drains, and wires connected to me to all kinds of ways. The only thing I could do was focus on things I love—my family, John Steinbeck, Aaron Copeland, Jim Croce, Grant Wood, and Thornton Wilder. I went through their works in my head.

What happened while I was asleep over those seven hours was pretty remarkable. They opened me up from my belly button to sternum. The surgical team removed my stomach, which apparently had tumors that spread from inside all the way to the outer lining. My spleen and a portion of my pancreas came next, because of their proximity to my stomach.

The esophagus and muscle around my stomach were tricky. They required a four-centimeter margin of healthy tissue to ensure that they had removed enough of my esophagus. Their first attempt did not achieve that, so they had to go in again. The team discovered microscopic cancer cells in the skeletal muscle in my ribcage and had to shave part of the muscle away to remove as much as they could. They could not guarantee that they had removed all of it. Essentially, they had scraped away a portion of my diaphragm. They inserted a feeding tube to finish things off.

When the dust settled, cancer was found in two of my lymph nodes but nowhere else, making it Stage 3A. It could have been a lot worse. But the mysterious microscopic cancer in my muscle that they couldn't ensure was gone left me worried.

The nurses found me a shared room by 11 p.m. that first night. Sharing a hospital room is among my least favorite things in the world, but the self-administered pumped Dilaudid kept me loopy all night. Plus, with a catheter in, there was no reason for me to even get up.

Based on remarks I overheard, I gathered that my roommate had the same cancer I had except two or three years ago, and they had just discovered a metastasized form of it behind his eye. This was not a good thing for him. I felt awful for him, but he was so loud that my sympathy was mitigated by annoyance. That's all I really remember from that first night. Becky, my angel, slept by my side in a chair. She had been there the whole time, along with my brother, mother, and other family.

At peak, I had four IV lines, three drains, one catheter, multiple electrodes, an epidural in my spine, a suction device inserted through my nose, and a breathing pump. I felt more like a robot or machine than a man.

The nurses tried their best, but the hospital experience is something I wouldn't wish on my worst enemy. Trying to unsuccessfully to pee with my heart rate jumping to

150, the young twenty-five-year-old nurses had to "straight catheter" me to empty my bladder. A suppository topped the experience.

I would wake up at 4 a.m. with horrendous diarrhea, sit naked in the bathroom, and have to wash myself with staples right up my middle like a zipper. The drains required constant maintenance and measuring of the fluid outtake. I felt reduced to a mere animal. I suffered through it, naked and cold, but strong in the bathroom as I washed myself off with a washcloth. I removed the old clothes, threw on the new, and got wired back up.

The drugs and environment created horrible nights sleeping. Cold sweats soaked my sheets. Sometimes nightmares invaded my dreams. I remember one where I told a colleague what doctor I was seeing and the hospital I go to and them looking at me like I'm so stupid. Others were incomplete memories where I remembered something, like a task, a letter or a grant request, not done, and I felt so sad and useless. I became aware of this constant sense of inadequacy.

This theme of inadequacy haunted me well beyond the hospital, as I relied on others for help and couldn't do the simplest things for months, even years. I would have these terrors that included fusions of all of my worries, roles, and responsibilities into one catastrophic scene. Finn's Cub Scout obligations, new exhibition gallery donors, and my newfound or newly rediscovered love of reading hardcore, real history books turned into stations that I was obligated to attend but considered skipping.

I dreamed of shooting a bunch of arrows into the sky and sending Finn out for a walk by himself while they rained down around us. I had sent out a friend to look after him from a high point to warn him if one was coming in close to him. What did that all mean? It sounds horrible.

The next two days were a blur. My lung almost collapsed after the first day. One by one, the tubes and devices slowly left my body, and I started feeling somewhat normal, but not without some craziness going down. I was just flesh and bones at that point. I woke up one night screaming about Lego Galaxy Squad because of an extremely heavy dose of Ativan mixed with Dilaudid. Exciting.

The days turned to a week, and I was getting restless. I wanted my home, I couldn't eat, and I was sick of rubber beds and mindless television. I finally returned home eight days after I arrived, but I was a different man. They had removed my whole stomach, entire spleen, a portion of my pancreas, part of my esophagus, and carved out suspicious-looking muscle in my chest cavity. The only thing sustaining my body was a bag full of formula that ran into a tube, into my jejunum for sixteen hours a day. My feeding tube.

There were humorous times in the hospital as well, believe it or not. The most ridiculous occurred at 1:30 a.m. on about night four. Becky was staying overnight, and I got up to use the bathroom, towing my IV line and feeding bag tower behind me. When I turned the light on, I saw a huge cockroach scatter across the bathroom floor. I instinctively, forgetting my post-surgery state, picked up a plastic urinal half-full of my own urine and, with all of my might, tried to smash the critter. I missed, and it took off into the room.

Bang! was all Becky heard, and she assumed I had fallen in the bathroom. She came rushing and called for nurses. Pretty soon, several nurses were in the room, all freaked out by the cockroach. I, incidentally, was okay.

"I know who we need," exclaimed one of the nurses. She ran off and found an eighty-year-old, feisty nurse assistant, who quickly grabbed a giant water bottle and chased after the roach like she was twenty-five. She found him and, with an uproar, successfully smashed him. I stood there speechless, urinal still dangling from my fingers.

By 3:44 a.m. on the day of discharge, I was obsessively preoccupied with my self-perceived inadequacy and worst fears of failure. How could I lay there in bed less than a week after all this started with *that* at the forefront of my mind? I should've focused on healing, family, and resting, and all I could think about was stupid work. I should've been thinking about Becky and the kids and surviving for them. I needed an about-face. I needed some positive thoughts. I needed some good dreams.

This whole time, I had not eaten, as all of my nutrition came through a feeding tube. At the end of day nine without food, food had become irrelevant to me. It's funny. I missed it, of course. But at the same time, I was not hungry and didn't crave anything. I just craved healing. I see commercials on TV for food and restaurants, but it seems like they were all designed for someone else, like a Lexus commercial, so I ignore them, even around Thanksgiving when every channel I turn on has some kind of special about cooking turkey or preparing stuffing.

Home, and Back Again

I finally made it home—thank God! I know that patience is one lesson from this. Another is probably an appreciation of the little things. For instance, why was my sense of smell so sharp? It was so strange. When I got home, I could smell things that I never could before and from much farther away.

This is like being born again, I thought. I appreciated the smell of food and drink, and I will soon appreciate small tastes of some things. When I'm all better but won't be able to eat large amounts of food, perhaps I will love tastes of things—a small bite of this, a sip of wine. *Maybe my sense of taste will be sharpened as well? I will certainly appreciate these sensations.*

Two weeks later, I found myself back in the hospital due to major dehydration. It was horrid. My wife had to drive me to the ER as I was shaking and mumbling to myself. We were stuck in traffic in the rain, two days before Thanksgiving, and I was on the verge of passing out on I-76 during rush hour. It took us two hours to drive fifteen miles to the hospital. We almost pulled over and called an ambulance, but I couldn't stand the insurance bill we would have gotten.

I spent my torturous first night back in the hospital in misery, pain, insomnia, and nausea. I prayed for ninety minutes straight through that night. I was alone. The only thing I could do was close my eyes and review my entire life with Becky from start to finish. Every little detail I could remember, I went through it all in my mind. The good times, the tough ones, love sparked, proposal, marriage, dogs we had, vacations we went on, commutes I had, homes we bought, kids being born, moving around so much, and living with her parents, twice. It's been nonstop love, passion, and also chaos.

Why can't we ever be nice and settled with a sense of normal? I thought. We had finally reached that when we moved back to West Chester with my good job, friends, school, and community. Now we had this, the ultimate chaos consuming everything. I'm so afraid that this will kill me. Not now, but not too far off in the future. How can I deal with this fear and not let it consume me?

That second week in the hospital was the most horrid thing I've experienced; much worse than the first time around, because that first time was a slow, gradual progress. The first week I endured twenty-five-year-old nurses shoving a catheter up my business at 3 a.m. when I couldn't pee, and others shoving suppositories, while getting pricked and poked on what seemed like an hourly basis. But I knew where I was heading—recovery and home.

But that second week was a total setback. I had an accident in my pants uncontrollably one night, like a baby. I spent Thanksgiving in the hospital alone, despite my family's best attempts to cheer me up with a visit. Every TV channel focused their program on turkey cooking while I couldn't eat. I didn't know what was wrong, why I was there, or when I'd go home. I lost ten pounds that week I would never gain back.

Finally, I came home again in early December with nothing really truly resolved. The only thing that seemed to help was that, after nearly three weeks, I could eat real food. That first bite of chicken noodle soup seemed to bring me back to life.

More Chemo and Proton Therapy

Then, things seemed to be in cruise control for a while. I was home with my family, gradually getting a little better every day. The feeding tube was still in full force, and as far as the doctors said, it would be there for a while. I woke up in the middle of the night, wandering around often, not able to sleep, then took long, deep naps during the day. I started chemo back up in January, having lost even more weight. My wedding ring dangled on my finger, and I was afraid I'd lose it. At my wife's suggestion, I switched hands to my beefier right-handed ring finger.

Later in the year, other things started to happen that indicated the same thing: I was withering away. My last belt loop wasn't enough for me to keep using the same belts. When I shaved, there were new concave sections of my cheeks that I had to carefully glide my blade over. It was unmistakable.

They said that this second round of chemo would be easy, and they were wrong. Every Wednesday for four weeks, I would get something called Folfox, another combination of drugs. After treatment in the office, I brought home a little ball-like pump with me. That pump hooked right into my port for two more fun days of chemotherapy action. It hit me hard. I felt depressed. It got cold outside. The side effects of chemo include a jarring electro-shock feeling in your extremities when subjected to cold. I dealt with this through February, rested for a month, and then went into radiation.

For radiation in the spring, the doctors said proton therapy would have less short and long-term side effects. Amazingly, you can get cancer from the regular radiation used to treat cancer! Since I was so young, they wanted to use the more targeted proton therapy, which must have cost a fortune. Five days a week for six weeks, I trekked downtown for my therapy.

I had to eat the exact same thing every day before treatment or else my bowels might shift if I introduced a new food. That got old very fast. When I arrived, sometimes the machine broke down and it took hours to fix, while other times it worked fine and I was home quickly. I developed rashes and felt a little ill at first.

Throughout those six weeks there was another routine: getting hooked up to my man purse. It was a pump, actually, that looked like a purse. Every Monday morning the home nurse came to connect it to my port, load it up with a 5-FU cartridge, and changed the battery before I took off for my first proton blast. I kept it with me all week until Friday afternoon. The smells of heparin and alcohol were the worst parts. They made me gag each time. But I managed all six weeks to avoid absentmindedly walking away from the pump while it was still hooked up to my body. By that point, I was used to being hooked up to stuff in general.

It seemed like a breeze when I finished and got to ring a special bell at the end of week six. The radiation oncologist had always warned, however, that the side effects could sneak up on you. "And they are cumulative, so they're usually worse towards the end," he explained.

I thought I had radiation beat and was scot-free, ready to move on with my life and come back only for my quarterly visits. But then a week later, I was totally laid out. I could barely move, eat, crap, or sleep. The radiation nearly killed me. They hadn't warned me of *that*. They only said about two weeks to recover. Well, those two weeks later turned to, "Well, it could take four to six weeks for your body to recover." I got so bad they admitted me to the hospital, performed a $400 co-paid endoscopy, and declared me fit. I lost another ten pounds.

Gradually I got a little better. My weight was up and down, but I was alive, and it was about a year after my diagnosis. So who would I be to complain? I've not been the same since and never will be, but I was functioning.

All the while, I was waiting for my August 6th CAT scan. Becky and I hadn't told anyone, but my June CAT scan showed spots on my liver that hadn't been there before. The only way to know if they were cancerous was to wait and see if they grow. "Cancer likes to grow," our oncologist said, and they were too small for a biopsy.

We spent the entire summer convinced that the cancer had spread to my liver, which is pretty much the same as a stage four curtain call in metastasis terms. I couldn't think about it. It made me cry. But then August 6th came, and the doctor called. I held my breath, and she said, "We're okay."

Becky and I jubilantly freaked out, hugging, crying, and I could only happily whisper, "Thank you," to my oncologist before hanging up. I made it through all clear, and we all thought that was it. The whole family, it appeared, would ride off into the sunset with a happy "The End" sign appearing for us.

But that wasn't the end. By mid-fall I was cranking along, slowly getting better. A little lighter than I would have liked, but I was back to work part-time. I was productive, doing things that were somewhat normal. I could have a couple of beers with friends at a bar on a beautiful fall afternoon. I could go to a Phillies or Flyers game with family. Becky and I attended social events and parties. We always left a little early, but I could eat, drink, converse, and socialize with anyone at that point.

Then, all of a sudden on Christmas, over a year after my surgery, I had an attack the likes of which I'd never experienced. *It's always on the holidays that these things happen!* I spent Christmas night on the second floor of my in-law's house, writhing in a single bed, sipping water, throwing up, and missing everything downstairs. It got slowly worse over the coming weeks. This painful ailment, a combination of pain and nausea with vomiting, became totally unpredictable so I never knew if I could keep a meal down or not.

At home, I would sit at the dinner table starving, take two bites, and then have to leave. The only way to combat this was to walk around the house pacing for thirty minutes or doing something to keep my mind and body moving. In the worst cases, I would eat something or even just take a pill, then up to fifty minutes later uncontrollably retch and throw it up.

By spring 2015, I was just stuck in limbo. I was still cancer-free, which was amazing news and meant that I didn't need a scan for another six months. But it's been a wild last month too. Almost every day I throw up, and my weight is dropping like a stone.

Last Saturday the most traumatic instance was just trying to take Finn on an errand. I had to catch vomit in my mouth and gurgle to him that I needed to pull over. I drove deep into the Mrs. Mikes parking lot, and it all came up.

I explained to him, "Daddy's just fine, Finn, just a little sick." I wasn't just fine. But then I cleaned myself up, and we went on our merry way to buy him some Legos and get me some drugs from the pharmacist.

I lost more weight, from 138 pounds or so to 130. They sent out a home nurse to make sure I was properly hydrated, which I wasn't. So for about three weeks, they hooked my up to a saline pump for two hours each day to give me more fluids. My house turned back into a hospital ward, with a pole, a pump, bags of fluid, syringes, alcohol pads, and Sharpied containers everywhere.

That didn't work, and I got worse. I could barely eat anything but very small meals, and was miserable on the couch most the time. So finally, they sent me into the hospital for TPN—Total Perinatal Nutrition—feeding. TPN is when they inject food right into your veins. In order to start the process, they need to install a PICC line (like a port) into your arm and monitor your reaction to the drugs for several days to ensure your body doesn't flip out. That meant another trip to...yes, to the dreaded hospital. I couldn't believe it. Here, fifteen months after my surgery, I was packing up my bags for another week in the hospital, that dreaded place. My fourth visit in fifteen months.

The idea was that I was going to gain weight and overcome my mystery ailment that way. Magically, things would just fall into place and my system would kick back in again. I went along with it because I had nothing else to go on.

"How much weight do you want to gain?" they asked.

My eyes widened like a kid in an ice cream shop. "How about fifteen or twenty pounds?"

I nearly drooled at the thought of gaining that much weight. Usually, I got excited about a pound or two. The thought of gaining fifteen to twenty pounds was almost unfathomable to me.

"Really? Fifteen to twenty pounds?" I asked in disbelief.

"Yes," they said. "That shouldn't be a problem."

So I checked into the hospital the next week to get things started, to the tune $500 per day in co-pays. Why the hospital? They needed to slowly administer this IV feeding and monitor me very closely to make sure my body didn't freak out.

TPN, I would learn, required a PICC line ("peripherally inserted central catheter") through my bicep. Using a wire as a guide, they stuck a flexible IV line deep into one of my largest veins near my heart. I assume this is because the viscosity of the formula needs a hardy vein and not some wimpy one near the surface.

Picture this: I arrived to a shared room with barely enough space to maneuver my IV pole to use the bathroom. My roomie, who apparently was in for some minor surgery, was a twenty-something immature kid.

He blared the TV all night and yelled things like, "Shut the fuck up, Ma. I don't need your help," until his mother left. I honestly think he lived at home and liked having his own space for a few days with a team of nurses to wait on him instead of his mother.

The PICC "team" came in and quickly turned my room into an OR-like sterile room. They shot my right biceps with multiple syringes of Lidocaine and inserted a flexible steel rod into my vein, which traces the path for my eventual PICC line, which will stay deep in my veins indefinitely.

It hurt to bend my arm, but I got used to this new piece of hardware to contend with. When I finally made it home, I had a new ritual. Each night, I spent a half hour mixing an elaborate and very expensive formula and hooking myself up to a pump to inject this milky concoction deep into my body through the PICC line. Here's an assessment of my status, as if I had to do some diagnostics:

- My weight: 121.4 pounds on March 10, 2015. I had lost about fifty pounds at that point.
- Spirits: at an all-time low. I realized that we would have to cancel our trip to Disney—a magical trip we surprised the kids with on Christmas.

Eating has become a chore and a science, if I can even make it through a meal. I try to reach another 1,000 calories each day in addition to the 2,000 through TPN, but with limited success. I take a pill thirty minutes before eating and swallow 10 ML of "Carafate," which is supposed to soften the way for the food. I'm really not sure if either of these works, but I just do them anyway. Then I have to find some applesauce, pour three Creon capsules that are cracked open like eggs over the applesauce, mix, and then eat. Then I sit and cut my food like a kid into little tiny pieces. I take one bite at a time and then wait two minutes after each bite. I watch the clock. Then the minute I feel like I might have eaten too much, I stop.

To deal with the discomfort and avoid vomiting, immediately after eating I do the dishes, walk around the house, or clean something mindless up. I put so much work into getting those calories and don't want to lose it. These are all techniques I've learned and am still learning, because no one—doctors, nurses, surgeons, or oncologists—has any idea what's happening to my body. I've been scanned, X-rayed, and tested in all possible ways, and on paper, I'm fine. But in reality, I'm suffering almost as badly as after my surgery. I can't go out, drink beers with friends, or even share a meal with my wife for a date night out.

For me, over a year after my surgery and twenty months after I was diagnosed, I take approximately thirty to forty pills daily. The two-month recovery has dragged on to twenty, and I'm worse off now than I was six months ago. My body is an enigma that no doctor can understand. I vomit when I eat, and now I get calories at night through Total Perinatal Nutrition (TPN) straight into my veins. I get two thirds of my calories that way now, and I spend most of my days on the couch in pain and nausea. This is the lowest point for all of us, and we are at our breaking point—the entire family.

Finally, in June of 2015, nearly two years since my diagnosis and twenty months since my surgery, I am barely hanging on. I can only force very small amounts of soft food down, and hope it stays. I have no energy to do anything. I wake up at 4 a.m., completely nauseous, and wander around the house trying to feel better.

We received new information from some scans, which looked like I had a partial obstruction and other problems, which are now finally showing up diagnostically. I found a new surgeon, burgeoning with confidence and experience. Surgery is imminent, and I simply cannot wait.

This time, instead of baby Moses, I know that I need something more to get me through. I need to go in tough and emerge tough, because my body has wasted away to nothing. So instead of baby Moses in the basket, I picture myself as grown-up Moses leading the Israelites to freedom. Parting seas, escaping the Romans, and everything else that came with it; I want to be that Moses.

The Emasculation of Cancer

There is something intensely emasculating about being so sick. In the beginning one day, I was in such intense pain and frustration that I sat on the back couch uncontrollably sobbing. I knew that I shouldn't cry in front of Becky and the kids, but I couldn't move and I couldn't hold it back. My nine-year-old daughter Abbie laid down next to me and consoled me. She held my hand and hugged me and almost cradled me like a big baby.

Even the mere act of getting sick reaffirmed this sense of losing my manhood. I'm literally shrinking and losing power. Just a few weeks after diagnosis, I already lost close to fifteen pounds. And I was in very good shape before. Now I am weak and powerless.

I have nightmarish thoughts about being put in a situation where I need to defend my family. We're being mugged on the street, Becky's getting aggressively hit on at a restaurant or bar, or someone breaks into our house. And I'm powerless to do anything about it. I've lost my manhood.

On the other hand, sometimes when I'm in church or at a school function for my kids, my mind wanders. I wonder what I would do if an active shooter came into the room. My first reaction would be to get myself and my kids out of there. But then I think, *Wait, of all of the people in this room, I'm the one who should tackle that bastard. If he kills me, I'll probably just die a few years earlier than I would have from cancer. So it should be me—I should be the one who plays the hero. It would just be the natural order of things.*

I plot this attack out it out in my head. *If I'm behind him, I should either attack with a swift blow to the head with some kind of object or jump on his back and choke him, judo style. If I'm in front, I just don't know. A completely suicidal run at him? I couldn't just sit there watching it happen, but perhaps I'd stand a chance of getting at him just because it would be so unexpected.*

Back to my emasculation. I even feel impotent, and I have had my sex drive literally sapped from me. How can I think about sex or get aroused when the world is collapsing all around me? Just like a child, I really have no sexual drive and instead I'm driven by love and the sensation of feeling loved. I'd rather cuddle and snuggle while I fall asleep than make love. I am five years old.

By December, I've lost thirty pounds. I hope I don't sound pompous saying this, but I used to be so strong and powerful. Thick chest and bulging biceps at 170 lean pounds with a six-pack. Even at age 40, I looked and felt very good. I had a full head of hair.

Now, I've shriveled down to someone who looks like he's on a hunger strike. My shoulders are boney, muscles are thin, and even my cheekbones have sunken in. My hair is thinning.

I've lost my manhood. Will I ever get it back? It just occurred to me yesterday, almost six months in, that I might never be anywhere near the same, near the old me. And for the first time in my life, I worry that my wife will not be physically attracted to me anymore. I worry it will be a pity attraction.

Instead of being in the middle of things, I have to just sit by while the kids are yelling, and I can't even discipline them. I can't mow the lawn or do anything around the house. Even the way I walk, kind of hunched over, eliminates my manhood. Instead of being tall and erect and strong, I'm stooped and weak and skinny.

The not-drinking thing is kind of weird too. It makes me feel like a preteen. I can't recall going so long without alcohol, having gone almost two months at this point. I was at parties drinking ginger ale and water for two months. Then I realized I could have a beer or two a day and started gulping them down. Now, without a stomach, I could deal with about one beer before I was doubled over in agony. But that only lasted a short while, and twenty months later, I can't fathom the thought of alcohol.

The feeling of being scared, too, is emasculating. I feel like I should be ashamed for being scared because of all of the happy, rah-rah, "let's beat this" attitudes out there regarding cancer. I'm scared shitless. Does that make me less of a man? The media makes me feel like it. Everyone expects cancer patients like me to be eternally optimistic, which I try to project, but it's tiring and also disingenuous.

The gifts people give me, like lotions, snuggly blankets knitted by old ladies, oversized cozy socks, and pillows, add to the emasculating effects of this. The foods that I wanted to eat early on before I lost my stomach, like pizza and ice cream, revert me to a juvenile state as well. Sometimes I scoop whole handfuls of Pepperidge Farm Goldfish in glee. Even my kids are too old to really enjoy them. I'm dopey and unsophisticated. I once got so excited about having ginger ale (a full can!) and popcorn and staying up late!

When I finish my dinner and clean my plate of food, I turn to my wife and say, like my six-year-old son, "I did a good job, didn't I, honey?" while looking proudly at my plate.

"Yes, you did great, sweetheart," she kindly replies.

My kids go on a camping night out with kind surrogate dads who watch after them. These substitutes are stronger than me, manlier, and more of a father to them than I can be now. They help them with s'mores and teach them to shoot a bow and arrow. The proxy dads worry about their safety in ways that I can't, because I would become a liability.

I remember this from when my father was sick, having to take care of him in unfathomable ways. He reverted almost to an infant like state at age 54 where he couldn't even take care of his basic needs. God, I hope I don't reach that point.

Like before, sometimes I dream about having to defend my family. I imagine something going horribly wrong, an accident occurring, or perhaps someone just picking on them. I have nightmares of a break-in into my house and large men coming to rape my wife. I know that I'm powerless to do anything in any of these situations. I imagine that if I do, someone will punch me out, and I'll be too weak to do anything, and they could actually kill me with one simple blow. And my port is my Achilles heel. If they hit that, or I fall on it, it will pop out of my vein and then I'll quickly bleed to death.

I think about this all of the time—when I'm asleep, food shopping, or walking through town. I'm weak and powerless to defend myself or the people I love.

After surgery, in the hospital, the descent into emasculation is complete. I cannot do anything myself. I shit myself. I shuffle down the hallway holding the hand of a one hundred-pound nurse. I can't reach my opposite armpit with a stick of deodorant to apply it and retain my dignity. I need help, I need drugs, and I need permission to do things. I call for nurses in the middle of the night with the call button, like a child calling for Mom and Dad because of monsters under the bed. I sob like a baby when the simplest things don't go my way, like dropping the soap on the floor and realizing that I can't pick it up. I need to be pushed around in a wheelchair. I'm weak and emaciated and bony. I can't pick anything up. I have to ask everyone for help.

At the hospital, you become a body. You strip naked and become a thing, objectified. They can't help it. It's their job. They, sometimes twenty-five-year-old nurses who were born when I was in college, put suppositories in your ass and catheter you when you can't piss. Your heart rate rises to 155 beats per minute because you're trying so hard to piss and avoid the catheter. They encourage you to take a shit, fart, like a pejorative coach. They mechanically stick your veins without mercy and give you bruising shots in your leg or ass.

I'm so young. Everywhere I've gone, in any ward over the last few weeks, I am always the youngest. You see the frail, naked, pale, scaly ankles of old men beneath the curtain as they strip to get into their gowns. Ironically, seemingly as a slap in the face, several months later, after surgery, after losing my weight but not my hair, I sat on the toilet at looked down at my own ankles. They looked the same as those described above, skinny, pale, dry, and scaly. I've become one of them officially.

During my second treatment, I can barely type because my fingers are tingly and prickly. Each keystroke sends a small shock through my body. The hospital is the great leveler in the chemo ward. People of all backgrounds and economic persuasions gather in one spot for one reason. The only exception is age. I'm still the youngest.

Some days, early on, I completely and totally forgot I was sick for a while. It was an uncanny feeling, and I greatly wish for those days back now, every single day. Once at the museum, I forgot that I was a cancer patient until the twinge in my stomach started and the modicum of dizziness set in.

CHAPTER FIVE
The Drugs

Passmore Williamson was an abolitionist who became an overnight celebrity when he was arrested in 1854 for helping an escaped slave and her children get to freedom. In 2013, his prison visitors' book, owned by the Chester County Historical Society, received over two million votes, making it the most engendered artifact in Pennsylvania.

In vivid detail, this chapter will explore the many drugs that were prescribed to me during this process. Bordering on bizarre and ridiculous, one drug in particular took center stage during my treatment.

HOUSTON, we have a problem. It was fall of 2014, and the sweet smell of sycamore leaves crushed on our town's brick sidewalks filled the air. It was supposed to be my favorite part of the year, but something was on my mind. It was October 2014, almost five months since my last treatment, and I was slowly, gradually, at a snail's pace, feeling slightly better.

What was bothering me wass this: On Tuesday September 30, "Split," the smaller of the two goldfish, had died. We had recently introduced two snails into their tank in an effort to keep it clean. Instead, I think it backfired, and those invaders must have introduced some kind of a virus or something. It was clear as day that the goldfish was dead. We held a funeral in the yard.

In the back of my mind I thought, *Well at least there's still one more goldfish left*—"Lickety"—*for me to outlive.* Shortly after this, we saw Lickety struggling. As if it were an emergency rescue, we quickly removed him from the tank and gave him lots of fresh water. Damn snails. Remarkably, Lickety recuperated and lived a normal life. I felt a sense of relief. Then, the unthinkable occurred. I found Lickety stone cold dead, sunk at the bottom of the tank, a few days later.

My heart sank, as now the only pet I had to outlive was Hudson, our half-blind Pointer. It discouraged me to think that the challenge was over. I could die any day now, and I *would* outlive the goldfish. The goldfish were like a drug for me, keeping me on track when I looked at them. But they were nothing like the real drugs I encountered during my pharmaceutical odyssey over two years.

When you have cancer, it's like *carte blanche* for prescriptions. Anything goes as long as it makes you feel better. That may sound nice to people who don't mind a mellow pill every now and then, but it doesn't help as much as you think, especially when they're only slightly effective.

I guess I'd better start with the hard stuff that they give you in the operating room or at least before a procedure. I should admit something: Before I found out I had cancer, I actually enjoyed the dozen or so non-life threatening operations and procedures I'd had in my lifetime. There was kind of a thrill to the surgery. Everything from the anesthesia, the fussiness about the procedure, the skill involved, and expertise all intrigued me. Being in the middle of the table and waking up to the coddling didn't hurt. That was something that I always found fascinating. But now, after two surgeries and many procedures in the last twenty months, I'm done and never want to be in a hospital ever again.

The Propofol I always found fascinating. It's that white stuff they call the "Milk of Amnesia." It's what killed Michael Jackson, but they routinely give it for all kinds of procedures. The last time I had it, I woke up trying to identify Yankees fans in the operating room and gave them a real hard time. Other times I'm sure I was not nearly as pleasant.

The best was probably when I had my second of four total endoscopies. I was determined, for some funny reason, to try to fight the Propofol. So as they started administering it, I stared at my name up on the big scope TV that was soon going to provide a private view of the insides of my guts. It displayed my name up in the corner, "Lukens, Robert."

As I was fighting the effects the drug, I exclaimed to the doctors and nurses my revelation. "My name—up there on the screen—needed to stay," I mumbled to them. "It needed to live on, just like me." I was determined then and there that I was going to win this cancer battle so that name in the corner of the monitor didn't end up on some gravestone but instead was on other things: papers, articles, websites, kid's cards, and programs. It needed to be a living name in the present tense, in the active tense, not in the past tense.

To them, it must have been comical, because as I had that revelation, I blurted this out through the circular plastic stint in my mouth for their camera to go down. "See that name! That's my name, and I'm going to see it up there forever. I'm going to live!" To them it was probably, "Blah blah blah! Wah blah wah blah blah!" which then faded to nothing.

For home, they gave me Vicodin with Tylenol at the beginning. This was for the cancer pain, which was pretty intense as the days wore on. It was a nice mild sedative that gave good afternoon naps after working nearly a full day soon after my diagnosis and took away the tumor pain. It is still one of my favorites, and I never became addicted to it.

From the beginning, they had also prescribed me Ativan, which has the generic name "Lorazepam," to take as one or two tablets every six hours as needed for nausea. These became another best friend. The nurse assistant whispered, "They're good for taking the edge off, too, especially at bedtime." My eyes lit up, and I have been popping several per day ever since, for nearly two years, and still going. I've since learned that most people are prescribed these drugs for anxiety, and I can see why because when I don't have one for a while I start getting catastrophically anxious thoughts about losing my wife, my home, and my job.

At one point, they sent me home with a 'script for a Fentanyl patch. Yes, Fentanyl is the stuff the bad guys on the street lace with heroin to give the user a stronger high. Heck, I tried it once, a twenty-four-hour patch. My dreams were kind of weird, but the worst came at about hour eighteen when it really snuck up on me. I was at work, feeling quite good, and having a conversation with a trusted coworker. Suddenly, I forgot the English language mid-conversation. My heart started racing, and I was sweating profusely. I ripped it off my shoulder right there and then. We had to keep those patches up high, lest the dog or kids got them until properly disposed of. That stuff is dangerous!

Along the way, I developed blood clots near my port. I woke up one morning, and my arm had swollen up like a balloon, which was how we found out. The solution was yet another drug. That day, I had to learn to give myself shots in the belly with a blood thinner called Lovenox. It was freaky at first, but eventually I got the hang of it. Each package of about thirty self-dosed shots cost around $8,000, and this was one of the cheaper drugs I was on. I easily topped six figures in just treatments within the first six months. After surgery, I gave myself the shots in my leg and butt for six months at 4 p.m. every day, causing lots of unsightly bruises and scabs. Finally, I was through with that about eight months later.

After my surgery, we left with a menagerie of drugs to keep me from being nauseous or in pain. There was Compazine, Zofran, Tylenol, and others. The only way to administer them was by self-injecting them into my feeding tube. At one point, they put me on Ritalin for nausea. It didn't work. None of them did.

But the magic drug was Dilaudid, which is basically a form of morphine. I loved it and looked forward to it in my foggy, post-surgical haze. It was a highlight of every day. At first I had to shoot the red stuff using a big fat syringe into the feeding tube. Then, I got it in pill form.

Knowing how addictive this stuff was, I kept telling the doctors, "We can try something milder if there's something to take," and they repeatedly said, "No, if this is working then let's stick to it." I either took that at face value and believed what they were saying or would nod my head while thinking that they know just how screwed I am with this cancer thing. So I thought, *who really cares if I get hooked on this?*

Getting a prescription of Dilaudid was like getting access to the Holy Grail. It must be hand-written, signed, and conveyed to the pharmacist directly. I timed them out perfectly so as not to run out, and I feared when I would be cut off for my abdominal pain. I'm still on it, and I hate to say it, but I look forward to it every day. Every four hours, I get to have a small break from this horror of waiting until I get cancer next. I've now tried to scale back and even "quit" several times, but the pain comes and the voices of the doctors saying, "Don't worry about it, Rob," echo in my head.

Nearly a year after my surgery, I could officially admit to myself that I was addicted to Dilaudid. I tried hard to get off of it, but the pain and discomfort were unbearable, and it was the only thing that worked. At one point, I was down to just two pills a day, as I methodically weaned myself off of them. But the doctors don't seem to care; only my wife and I do. So why not just take as many as I need? Now I'm up to seven, and I'm ashamed. When I have a fresh new bottle of 150 pills, I'm secretly relieved. The one day I ran out was scary; going cold turkey is not recommended by anyone.

Now it has been a year and two months since my surgery, and I'm still totally addicted to Dilaudid. I'm plotting my way off of it, though. Like trying to quit smoking, I've tried to get myself off of it several times and went back due to some kind of a trigger. I was so close last spring, but then had my "dark time," which is what I call the two or three weeks I barely remember after my radiation when I was like a zombie. I've been taking them pretty much full time, as much as I can during my waking hours, ever since. The nurses and doctors still nicely say, "If you need it, if you are in pain, then do not feel bad about taking it." That doesn't help me in my quest for normalcy, though. I'm conflicted, as I do need something because I'm in pain and discomfort all of the time. But I feel like it owns me now. I count the hours until I can take the next one.

I am now on my third time trying to quit this drug, which I'm convinced has something to do with my less-than-stellar recovery. At one point, I was up to taking 20-24 mg a day, which is like popping as much as I could non-stop. Part of it was the pain I was trying to get rid of, the rest was this hollow feeling that the Dilaudid exterminated for a couple of hours. I thought I was onto something, though. *Is the Dilaudid (essentially morphine) causing the pain when I don't have it? Like a self-fulfilling prophecy?* I think so.

I've cut my consumption by more than half, and I'm on Day Two of one of my cut back days. I just reduced the amount I take by 33 percent, and I am going through intense withdrawal. I didn't realize that if I reduce my dosage once a week by 2 mg, which was my plan, eventually the cut would be exponentially more. I can barely keep my mind straight and can barely type this right now. To distract myself, I jump from one activity to another like a flea. I do dishes, work on my computer, dust the house, and put stuff away that's been out for weeks.

It's the oddest, worst feeling, and I need to beat this once and for all. Just goes to show what a hold this has had on me for eighteen months! I can only imagine what it's been doing to my mind and body. I know I've been snappy with my wife and kids and distracted at work, but I'm also in intense pain, too, and only the Dilaudid takes care of that. But not anymore.

The first time I tried to get off the narcotic, I tried cold turkey because I ran out of pills, and it was *hard*! I felt like I was just dying coming off of these pills. At 4 a.m. one night, I realized I could only sleep for a couple of hours at a time, then drift off, then wake up abruptly. And there was no end in sight. The next day was the worst day. Stomach pains emanated throughout my whole body. I was trying to hang on and think of the other side—life without narcotics. But it's so damn hard. My body shakes, and I feel like every muscle needs to be super stretched, every joint cracked.

A few days later I realized that there was no way to do it cold turkey. But I still found myself at 3:30 a.m., slugging back a glass of white wine and an Ativan on the couch, watching late news, trying to go to sleep. I was desperately seeking sleep. *Why does it all of a sudden elude me when it came so easy a week or two ago?* Pure, blissful sleep. I was sleeping ten hours a night, waking up just once to piss. Now it was a battle that I had to plot out all of a sudden. I timed the Ativan, stretched my body beforehand, toss and turned, while trying not to wake anyone up. Finally, I realized that I had a few Vicodin saved from before my surgery. They were huge horse pills, so I used a mortar and pestle to grind them up to swallow. Finally, narcotic relief. My prescription for Dilaudid arrived the next day, and my first attempt was over.

Another time, I tried to wean myself off it of it about nine months after surgery, and I got down to two total pills a day, which was a huge deal. But then I checked in with all of the nurses and doctors and asked what I could use to replace it. There were no solutions or any encouragements to get off of it. So I said, *forget it, I'll take it and it alone as long as it works, and I won't feel guilty about it.* In fact, my oncologist said, "Don't worry about it—whatever you need to stay comfortable." I've stuck to her philosophy ever since, which is basically returning to six to eight Dilaudid pills a day.

So in April 2014, eighteen months after my surgery, I was still taking this stuff. I think it made me skinny. I looked like one of those opium addicts from old nineteenth century sketches, or a POW. I looked into a mirror, and all I saw sometimes was a skull coming through my skin staring back at me. I lost so much weight.

This time, I'm determined to beat it, though. I've tried everything before. Once, I told my wife to hide them and dole the white pills out gradually to wean me off of it. But I broke down, and it didn't work anyway because the doctors and nurses kept reassuring me, "If you need it, take it!" I can still hear it in my head.

Then I had a major setback in the winter of 2015, as I went back into the hospital with major malnutrition and weight loss. I was down to almost 120 from an original 170 pounds. I hate everything about being in the hospital: the sticky rubber beds; the smell of urine, vomit, and shit through the halls; the constant waking up in the middle of the night for changed IV bags or blood samples; and the loneliness. It makes me literally cry to think about going back, and I will do anything to not be in the hospital.

When I got out of the hospital, with a little encouragement from my wife, I decided that this time, it was just me and the stuff, going head-to-head. I decided to beat Dilaudid. I had been on it for eighteen months! And before that, if you include the Vicodin, it had been nearly two years of constant narcotics!

This newfound drive gave me a competitive prize to really focus on—something totally in my control, really, when there was so much that wasn't. And I don't ever want to go back into the hospital. I want to gain weight, feel right, and move on. So I started with four pills, and gradually by halving a pill every week, now I'm down to two. I get itchy all over, antsy, upset, and depressed as I experience withdrawal, but I work my way through it mostly by distraction and looking forward to the next pill. Sometime there won't be a next pill or even a half pill, but I will be even stronger when I'm there in a few weeks. So far, I go to the gym, walk circles around the house, and write this, and it keeps me focused on other stuff when I'm literally itching for more Dilaudid.

I feel like I am in the darkest hell right now. 4 mg of Dilaudid left per day. Down from 20 mg per day six weeks ago. Only two weeks until I am free of this demon, which I now crave like a vampire craves blood. G. Raymond Rettew never had to deal with this—a battle against a full-blown addiction to morphine.

There were other drugs, too, for pain, constipation, radiation burns, indigestion, etc. I took, and still take, Pancreon enzymes so I actually digest my food, since I have half a pancreas. There were also wounds to manage, such as my feeding tube, which formed a new scab each day, and the drains that seeped orange and pink fluids out of my thorax just after the surgery. I had to measure the daily output from the drains for the first few weeks. Later in the process, they tried everything to deal with the nausea. First they tried Gabapentin, which is supposed to heal nerve endings but also help with seizures and bipolar disorders, and then the Ritalin. Neither helped. The way I saw it, it was just me and this illness doing battle, and I needed to will my new body to work with the aid of as few drugs as possible.

Back to the feeding tube, which clogged from time to time and required ginger ale or cranberry juice to free the seized formula. The first time this happened I cried because I thought it meant a trip to the ER. Instead, a home nurse, God bless her, took two hours to free it, and the contents of the tube—Coke mixed with half-digested food—shot across the room with a lot of force. I got really good at unclogging my feeding tube, which was still inside me six months after my surgery. The worst thing about the feeding tube was that my nightly feedings left me smelling and sweating an awful sweat. That smell was awful.

The sensation of being attached to something, like a feeding tube or IV line, never fully left me. Five months after they removed the tube, I walked into the bathroom and my iPhone was in my pocket with headphones on. The headphones caught on a doorknob and popped out of my phone, and I gasped in horror, almost doubling over in anticipated pain and discomfort. I thought my feeding tube had popped out, stitches and all, even though it had been gone for months!

Towards the one year mark, entirely too late in the process, we were introduced to Marinol or "Dronabinol," as they call it in the pharmaceutical world. Unfortunately, we found it too late for when I needed it most during those super dark weeks when I was a zombie. I could take one of these, basically pot in pill form, every four hours if I really wanted to. It is THC, the active ingredient in pot, suspended in sesame oil. But taking it all of the time would turn me into a total wastoid, because nothing would ever get done. I wouldn't shower, talk, write, or function at all. But I laughed and ate a lot the few times I took it. Sometimes, however, it turned sinister, and you could really lose your shit. One time, about an hour in, I was crying like a baby about what a failure I was and was becoming. Becky calmly talked me down, saying that I was super successful and didn't have to worry about losing my job. This thought about losing my job was a constant and totally irrational worry, though, with Marinol or not.

Most potent drugs like Marinol give you warnings about not operating equipment or vehicles while on them, and I now heeded all of these warnings, specifically within the first hour when they usually took effect. However, the first time I took Marinol, I was totally blindsided.

Somehow, I missed the "time release" aspect of those little rubber-looking footballs filled with THC. So an hour and a half after taking my first one, I figured I was fine, so I drove the kids to the Walgreens pharmacy just six blocks down the street.

Between the time when I left and I arrived, in those three minutes, I became a different person. I arrived completely stoned. In fact, I pulled into a parking spot, thought I saw a bee's nest in front of the car, warned the kids, and immediately moved the car a few spaces away in about a five- to seven-point turn. All of that must have looked hilarious on a security camera. Somehow I got through picking up my next 'script, while the kids perused games and toys, and drove home slowly at ten miles per hour under the speed limit while hugging the white line on the right side of the road. From that point on, I knew those pills were special and nothing to mess with.

My tactic, as I continue in my quest to divest myself of Dilaudid, is to use a lower half dose of Marinol to help. This can be used, I decided, to help wean me off of the real morphine. We will see how that works. All I know is that I have to do something. I literally take 30-35 pills a day. It's insane, and I know it has to contribute to my depression, feeling like I'm trapped in this body, and inability to gain weight.

CHAPTER SIX
The Things People Say and "Journeys"

Bayard Rustin was a civil rights leader and right hand man of Martin Luther King, Jr. He was also gay, and because of that, his many accomplishments were relegated to the background of the movement. He recently posthumously received the Presidential Medal of Freedom in 2014. He was also from West Chester.

The chapter will focus on people's reactions to cancer and how ludicrous they usually are. This includes everything from "close friends" who never sent a card or placed a call to those who were almost strangers and saved the day numerous times or selflessly gave themselves over and over again. This chapter will be filled with ridiculous examples, heartwarming stories, and a literal how-to react to and support people with cancer and what to and what not to say. This will also include all of the advice received, acupuncture, and failed and humorous attempts to find an adequate cancer-oriented therapist.

WHATEVER you do, reader, please learn this next point from this book. Cancer patients, at least this one, want your love, your support, and your understanding. But we really don't want your advice. We shun your stories about how great your life is. And most of all, we rarely want to hear your own struggles with cancer or any other illness, or the struggles of a loved one.

From Day One, the comments that came out of people's mouths about my cancer were shocking. I was given all kinds of advice. Many people compared my cancer struggle to their own. "You'll be just fine," they said. "I would just get my radiation on lunch break, and it was just an inconvenience." Echoes of John Hope Franklin rang through my ear. Many others shared these same sentiments, telling me I'd be tough and I'd undoubtedly be fine soon. They did not realize what a formidable opponent my cancer and treatment schedule would be.

Others talked of parents or even grandparents who beat this or that cancer. Some didn't even compare my challenge to cancer at all. One person tried to tell me he could relate because of heart trouble and how gut wrenching it was to learn that he might have to give up jogging. Who cares? Not me. I just want to live a somewhat normal life, and could give up jogging or just about anything else to get there.

I had what one good friend called "funky cancer," and no one seemed to understand that except me and the medical team. That team sometimes looks at me as if I should have died by now because of how bad it was and how extensive my surgery was.

The pressure to be strong and appear like you have it all together is pervasive for cancer patients. You get it from friends and family trying to be encouraging. It appears even more when you look at commercials, campaigns, and the go-get-'em attitude of cancer speakers and the media. That's all you hear from these outlets: perseverance, grace, and overcoming the odds.

This is a fantasy. There's no mention of the vomiting, the blood, the diarrhea and constipation, or the fatigue that makes you feel less than human. They don't mention the dangers of a drug addiction that comes with cancer. I cannot imagine anyone going through what I've gone through and keeping a positive attitude 24/7. Where's the reality of this?

On TV, they talk about treatment plans, "So you can fight your cancer and never miss a beat." They show "a celebration of sisterhood, of love and life" for cancer survivors running half-marathons. "The cure is within," another cancer patient states as he appears to have defeated metastasized lung cancer. The instances of celebration and the seeming inevitability of cancer survival are abundant.

I've even heard of an organization for young adults with cancer that tries to make cancer seem like no big deal. The organization's website shows young people clapping as if they're in a fundamentalist church, and there are pictures of galas and conferences on their site. But my least favorite image is a photo of women in bikinis and bare-chested men holding drinks like they're on spring break. They're trying to make cancer look cool and beating it even cooler.

This positive image has been fabricated for several reasons. In an altruistic sense, I suppose they are trying to inspire people like me. But then there's also the fundraising needs for those institutions that need the money and need to show successful battles against cancer. Finally, it makes for great newsworthy human-interest stories that suck people in.

Instead, what these resources really make me want to do is throw a shoe at the TV. We see pink cleats on football players. There are infinite walks, runs, concerts, tweets, celebrity cancer announcements, and even music videos, but what's missing is the pure anguish of total pain and nausea that is unsolvable and may never go away. What's missing is facing the possibility of death and not feeling like you've adequately lived your life or provided for your family.

This whole positive cancer movement also attacked my manhood. If I couldn't be positive, be a leader, or shrug off cancer—as one commercial claimed, by easily just "riding my bike to and from therapy"—then what kind of a man could I be? Pairing this with my inability to care for my family and work, I was thoroughly emasculated. I can't pick up my son—my wife has to do that when he's fallen asleep in our bed. I can't take them to Disney World or snowboarding, let alone walk across town to get gelato. I'm a shell of a man. Where is that in all of the cancer-oriented public relations materials?

I don't mean to sound completely negative about this. Yes, we need inspiration. And there are many good organizations with good messages that *do* inspire and help people. What I am criticizing, in a nutshell, is the wholesale glorification of cancer struggles and survival as some epiphany-like life journey, like taking an Outward Bound class or doing an Iron Man competition.

Stupid Things People Say

Let's get back to my original intent: the stupid things people say. These are legion, but here are some of the top ones that stand out and hurt the most:

- When we asked one of the surgeons who we saw early on how I could have gotten cancer, he said, "Do you eat a lot of lunch meat? Ham? Bacon?" On the way out of his office, he nonchalantly said, "There is a sign-up sheet to schedule your stomach removal for next week." This was less than a week after my diagnosis.

- The first email from someone I hadn't talked to in years: "Oops, looks like you have a road bump on the road of life to overcome!" A "road bump"—really!?

- In addition to the direct hits like this, there were the people with the insensitivity to send all of the details of their trips to amazing places. "We just returned from a trip to Tahiti," one went on, "and in a word, it was *fabulous*!" The closest thing we had to a vacation at that point was a room in the hospital with a sweeping view of the city.

- When meeting with one doctor's interns preparing for the next phase of this hell—radiation—we had to painstakingly rehash the entire the history of these last few months. When the doctor realized that I had a total gastrectomy, she looked at us and asked, "Well, how do you eat without a stomach?" She wouldn't let it go, saying, "I mean, really, how do you actually eat?" Shouldn't she know that?

- Walking into a doctor's office and having him immediately blurt out so all can hear, "So how did they find it? Was there pain? Were you throwing up? Did you have bloody diarrhea or something?"

The ultimate, however, was from a family friend. I had purposefully kept my illness off of social media and asked friends and family to do the same. Why? I felt that it made light of a very serious situation.

On the morning of my surgery, during all of the uncertainty and anticipated pain, someone broke the rule. He posted on Facebook: "Pray for Rob, who has stomach cancer and is having his stomach removed today." The kicker is his very next line jubilantly announced he was getting new household appliances. He was getting new appliances while I was having my stomach removed—the magic of social media. The post was eventually removed.

Some family sent postcards from beautiful places, while others were sensitive enough to not even tell me they were going away. Friends group-texted pictures of paradise while I wasn't even well enough to take my kids to Disney or out to breakfast. I missed about 150 different social events in West Chester on an annual basis and heard about them too. Gone were the invites to poker nights or happy hours—I guess they knew better.

My wife has her own list that she keeps track of, as she gets it just as much as me. "What is wrong with people, seriously?" we agree.

Here are some of hers:

- In conversation with someone during the height of surgery and chemo, this person actually said how exhausting it was to deal with an extended family member enduring radiation for cancer.

- During a cardiologist appointment for stress and heart pain, she described how the cancer stress is affecting her, and the nurse exclaimed, "I completely understand. I have had to pop a few Xanax myself because I am planning my wedding right now, and it is *so* stressful." She was older than her, and a nurse! She should have known better.

- When talking to someone about my sickness and how I lost weight and looked different, they commented, "Well, he still looks good, not quite like a Holocaust victim." This came up again a month later, this time saying that I was now too thin and would be a perfect fit for a role in a Holocaust movie, if given the chance.

- Among friends one day, when she was talking with the women who should understand and show support, one woman complained about her husband who refused to take out the trash by saying, "It's not like he has cancer." I don't think we have ever once argued over who was going to take the trash out.

Most people are naturally unreal, we decided. They are naturally so self-absorbed and stuck within their own thoughts and lives that they don't even have a clue what their stupid dribble sounds like to someone in a crisis who's screaming for help and companionship. Luckily, we knew that we could replace every one of those foot-in-mouth comments with hundreds of loving, thoughtful, heartfelt words that still bring tears to my eyes. It's just that the misplaced comments hurt a hundred times worse than the kind gestures could ever feel good.

Another thing that we've noticed is that the word "journey" is everywhere. Everyone who has cancer, apparently, has a cancer "journey." This is part of the rhetoric of cancer, and it is pervasive. It elicits images of someone walking through a path in the Tulgey Wood of Lewis Scott Carroll's *Jabberwocky*, or someone triumphantly climbing Mount Everest, just like they will inevitably overcome the cancer beast.

I detest the phrase "cancer journey" because for most, or at least me, it's a not a journey. It's a scary real life nightmare full of ambiguities, pain, and the real possibility of death. I wouldn't compare it to anything but a terrifying nightmare of epic proportions, which negatively affects every aspect of your life. Except this nightmare is real, and cancer is the devil.

Therapists

From the beginning of my treatment, we had a bubbly social worker available to us. Usually, she arrived in our chemo room at the most inopportune times. With my eyes closed, soaking in chemotherapy and trying to sleep, she would knock-knock and come on in to ask how we're doing.

I'm sitting here, at age 40, with poison being injected into my veins to keep me alive, I would think, *how do you think I'm doing?*

She'd ask about the kids, even though she clearly didn't have any, and then would disappear until my next treatment. Later on, she suggested cancer-oriented psychotherapy, and I actually agreed with her. I could use someone to talk to.

This therapy thing is a tricky one. I actually snuck into the therapy thing through the back door, and well before the social worker suggested it. It started with a group session through "guided imagery," which I believe very much in. That's when you get several people together, and you have a leader (the therapist), and she relaxes you and almost hypnotizes you into thinking about happy thoughts that address your fears and thoughts and challenges related to cancer.

I enjoyed guided imagery immensely and even tried it on my own. But the first time I did it, I ended up imagining myself in our kitchen in Wilmington, where we had lived three years back. I could hear our children's laughter in the background as they rambled through, with familiar fruit smells wafting the air. In my case, that smell was tangerine. I snapped out of the trance bawling, literally in front of a room full of strangers. There were no tissues nearby, so I wiped my snot on my sleeve, hoping that everyone still had their eyes closed.

The second time was magical, at that same exact session. I imagined I was in Utah or something like it. I was surrounded by flat red rock. I had a "journey" to make and just knew that I had to move forward along this smooth, dry river of red rock. I walked confidently, and when I reached a certain spot, there was a man there. Wearing a backpack, he was propped above me on a four-foot ledge of rock. The therapist was later impressed that I had found a "spirit guide" in my vision—a person to help me.

This guy was my savior. He was about forty-five, not clean-shaven but no beard, and he knew where we were going, even though I didn't. There was somewhere to go from there, he motioned, and I needed to follow him. He reached down and grabbed my hand in a manly way, reaching around my wrist. He was proud of me and of my resolve and encouraged me to continue on. He pulled me up and told me to follow him. I did just that. And then I came to, my eyes dry and a smile on my face.

That man, with his scruffy face, tough-looking outerwear in a red pull-over shell, was confident and comforting. He has been in my thoughts ever since this vision in Summer 2014. I seek him out and know he doesn't exist in the real world, but I find elements of him in people. I find him in people that have had "funky cancer" and get it. I find him in good, selfless friends who follow through and care. And I have found that I find him in Jesus Christ.

My other sessions with therapists have not been so successful. I did have one session with the woman who ran the guided imagery session, and she was great. She listened, a rare and important thing, and acknowledged what a shitty card I was dealt. She had some great ideas about getting others to understand this and that my whole cancer battle wasn't really "over," ever.

Then, due to insurance, I had to find a new therapist to help me reframe my life in light of my diagnosis and recovery. That was my goal, very clear: reframe and refocus.

Finding that therapist, however, seemed impossible. Insurance didn't cover most plans, and co-pays were high. So I had to really dig deep and search. I talked with many people and met with others. Finally, I met a kind of shrink broker who would place me with the right person. He was kind of like a triage nurse at an ER.

It did not go well. I received a call a week later from potential shrink number one, and it was a shock. First, he called me to set up an appointment while he was driving in his car when he couldn't even look at his calendar. That didn't make sense, and I decided I could overlook this if we could even get an appointment set up.

But then the shrink started to probe. I imagined that he was driving a Prius down the freeway while eating a Big Mac and drinking a giant Coke, too.

He said, "I know your case, and I'm not scared away." He cited numerous cancer cases in his family, which I suppose made him qualified.

To this, I responded that I was surprised that he would even say such thing, as I thought doctors such as he were supposed to listen to clients first.

Instead of listening to me and to my situation, the shrink continued by saying, "I bet you have regrets. Everybody does," as he darted down the highway with the imagined burger in hand.

At that point I knew things were going awry. I assured him, "I have no regrets, and I am solely focused on the future and being a good husband and dad, both now and in the future."

But he persisted, insisting that I must have regrets by saying, "If you are that clean, you're the first person I've ever seen without regrets." He assured me that he would help me understand my regrets that I was not aware of.

From there I told the doctor that it might be best for him to listen to me talk for a little bit at our first session and to determine what I needed. To which, he swung back to these hidden regrets that I inevitably had. We made an appointment, and then I canceled it five minutes later.

The triage man called later and apologized profusely. He said, "I will help find the perfect person for you, Rob."

I received another call a few days later from shrink number two, and I pulled into her parking lot a few weeks later. After struggling to find a secret, unlocked door near the loading dock, I finally entered her office on a dark, snowy evening.

I was hopeful this time. Perhaps this one could help me frame this new approach to a new lifestyle as a cancer survivor and post-gastrectomy patient, and all that came with that. Instead, she appeared to know nothing of cancer or working with patients with cancer.

The moment I knew that this was another big mistake came three minutes in. When asked about my profession, I told her I ran a museum. She nonchalantly asked me the most offensive and ear-piercing question that I encounter on a semiannual basis: "So you must have another job, then, right?"

The implication of this frequent question is obvious. The question really is, "This is not a serious enough career, so you must pump gas to make ends meet, right?"

I reassured her that I had a Ph.D. in American History, twenty people working for me, and required no second job. I immediately checked out of the conversation for the next fifty minutes.

So that left me therapist-less and content to just move on without one, to be frank. At that point, it was more stressful to try to find one than it was worth.

Meanwhile, my wife was on the prowl for a good person to talk to about the stresses of being the wife of a cancer patient. As she should. She got the last therapist left in a firm nearby that specializes in such things—cancer, trauma, death, etc. When I called a few days later, they ironically had no room for me.

CONCLUSION
Jesus Is An Intrepid Explorer

Sam Entrikin *was second in command of Robert Peary's 1893-1894 expedition to the North Pole. His story is riveting and the stuff of Hollywood. He barely made it out alive, and I've thoroughly researched his correspondence and diaries. Ultimately, Entrikin, also of West Chester, saw himself as a new American man. With the supposed closing of the American frontier, the Arctic provided the best new frontier for proving one's manhood. From how he used facial hair to how he endured many repeated hardships, Sam provided inspiration for me during my most difficult days.*

The man with the backpack is a combination of all of these extraordinary historical men, whose stories helped me through this difficult ordeal. This chapter will wrap it all together, and the man with the backpack is someone I encountered during a mindfulness cancer session whom I believe represents God. I thought of him often but never met him, but I believe he was with me the whole way. I encourage readers to find their own man with a backpack to lead them through this experience and help them through the wilds of cancer life.

REMEMBER the guided imagery and the man with the backpack? I continued with this guided imagery on my own often, when I needed inspiration.

When I closed my eyes, I relaxed and went to that Utah desert, red, solid rock surrounding me on all sides. I elaborated on the scene, imagining cool blue pools of water scattered about here and there. I hiked or sometimes biked with a super-strong, healthy body—the body of a man in his twenties. Heck, the body of my forties before my cancer D-Day. In this place, I was alone.

I could swim naked. I could run, jump, and rest to absorb the vista around me. I would get lonely, though, and knew I needed a companion—no, more like a guide. So I would seek the man with grizzly stubble, the man with the backpack I met before, to show me the way.

I find him each time and, wordlessly, we exchange greetings and admirations. He is about my age, maybe a little older, maybe a little younger. He knows where to go and what to do.

Because I felt like there needed to be a destination, I thought of a plateau, like the big one in Australia. He led me there once, sometimes pulling at my arm or hand. We walked, and I felt the bits of orange stone crush beneath my feet. I loved the feel and sound. We made it to the top, and there the plateau actually hugged me, somehow. There were places to sit and feel the warmth of the sun and lie against rock-hard stones that were as comfortable as a bed. I could see forever.

Back in the real world, an epiphany came to me. My Ph.D. dissertation in American History was all about Arctic exploration, and here I am on my own hell of a challenging trek, not "journey," to defeat cancer and resume some sense of normalcy. My Arctic explorers endured incredible things. Some lost toes after hundreds of miles in search of the North Pole. Others resorted to cannibalism to survive another winter. Still others were trapped in the ice for years until deciding to move on their own in search of civilization over 600 miles away. Scurvy, walruses, ice floes, starvation, and sinking ships all posed dangers at every turn.

So here I am, a hundred years later, in the middle of this struggle that parallels the experiences of those men. I can't turn back and need to go on.

And I have decided that the man I need to get me there, wherever there may be, is Jesus. Only, he's not a carpenter in robes or bearded and on the crucifix. He's a mysterious mountain guide. The end might be life for another twenty years with my wife and kids, or it might just be dying with a purpose and a plan. That's all I want, Jesus mountain guide, a purpose and a plan to die, if that's Your will.

This is all very comforting to me, and I want more of it. This is the answer. Jesus won't make stupid comments about cancer, he will not call only to ignore me because he's scared of cancer, and he won't ask me if I needed another job to care for my family.

I was worried for a while about church and God and all of that for a number of reasons. Some were practical, like where would my service be held if I was buried? How else would Becky have a support group if I died? Others were more self-serving, because I believed in God and wanted to raise a godly family. I also wanted to make sure that they grew up in such an environment. Plus, if I died, the best place for Becky to find a new husband would be at a good, supportive church.

If you take the characteristics of these other men who inspire me—Fred Shero, Sam Entrikin, Passmore Williamson, G. Raymond Rettew, and so on—the grit, resolve, and perseverance they showed are all characteristics that

I believe will help me beat cancer. It will not be flashy websites or marathons that will get me better. There will be no commercials or *Today Show* episodes of inspiring stories that will help me. The friends who never call while they know I suffer won't inspire me. I turn to history, and first and foremost, Jesus Christ, my man with a backpack.

To do this, to turn to him, I close my eyes, put on gentle music, and go back to the red rock desert. I yearn to see him, to feel the comfort of his blue-eyed gentle gaze, and follow him to the end. There, perhaps I'll find my father, perhaps I'll find normalcy, I don't know. All I know is that, in all of this senselessness, following the man with the backpack is the only thing that makes sense.

The End

FINDING STRENGTH AND GOING HOME
By Rebecca Lukens

ROB met that man with a backpack on August 1st around 11:30 p.m., surrounded by his family at home. He went very peacefully without a sound; his heart just stopped. It is a day I will never forget.

After months of trying to figure out what was going on and why he was still so sick, spitting up bile constantly and losing more weight, we knew we had to do something by June. By then he was so uncomfortable and could hardly even sleep. It was all so puzzling. All of his scans were good and showed no signs of cancer. It was decided that surgery was the best option so they could perform what they said would be a "mechanical fix." We were so hopeful and even told the kids, "Daddy is going to go in, and they are going to fix this little issue and then he is going to be better and get stronger." The surgeon was to reroute some of the connections made during his first surgery and move the bile duct down lower so he hopefully wouldn't be spitting bile into a cup every few minutes, sometimes seconds. He went in for surgery on June 11th, and it was then we were told very grave news: The cancer had spread in several places and was inoperable. I was the first one to talk to him while he was recovering from a surgery that hadn't happened and still foggy from the anesthesia. When I walked in the room, he knew something was wrong just from the look on my face. But what was so hard was trying to tell him what I had just been told an hour ago, the words reverberating in my head like a bouncy ball, three to six months, three to six months. I somehow had to tell him the cancer had come back, and I had to tell him it wasn't good. It was so awful, but then he asked me how long he had to live, and I couldn't answer. I just cried. He asked, "A year?" I shook my head no, and he asked, "Nine months?" When I shook my head no again, he asked, "One to three?" I told him no and then he asked, "Three to six?" I shook my head yes and just cried and held him. We had just been given his death sentence.

I'll never forget, while he sat still in that hospital recovering from the attempted surgery, I somehow had to wrap my head around taking Abbie and my niece to a Taylor Swift concert. The tickets had been purchased months earlier for a birthday gift, and we had splurged and gotten her floor seats. With everything else, the thought of not going with her would have been so devastating. I will never forget standing there watching her, her innocent face, having the time of her life, while I stood there constantly thinking that in a few short months her dad, my husband, might not be here. I stood there with thousands and thousands of fans, trying to enjoy myself for Abbie. I cried almost uncontrollably at one point when Taylor Swift started talking about the empowerment of woman and being strong and if that wasn't enough, Rachel Platten came out and sang "Fight Song." That was it. I was a mess, trying as hard as possible to hide my tears as I listened to this song that has been so inspirational for so many and thinking, *How in the world am I going to do this? How will I be strong?*

We still hadn't told the kids anything at this point yet. Telling the kids that the cancer had come back would be even more excruciating, harder than the first time. They were eleven and eight and had been through so much already in their young lives. This time we knew so much more, and our hope was being crushed. He was able to leave the hospital a couple of days later, but we weren't going to let this be the end. We still held on to hope and made as many connections, phone calls, emails, and plans to start chemo and a possible clinical trial as fast as we could.

That was our mission for a few weeks until it all stopped short. I had to race him to the ER, and after some tests, they discovered a blockage. He was transferred to the city during the middle of the night. The whole next day, we waited for them to wheel him back for emergency surgery, until they told us what we didn't want to hear: It was too dangerous. It just got worse. We were told very abruptly he only had days to a week to live. We thought, *What? How is that possible, this death sentence closing in even more?* We were shocked, sat in disbelief, and asked how this was happening. He's here only a few more days? We had our pastor come down, and as we prayed, he spread oil on his forehead. Rob and I had those conversations you only can have when your life is being stolen away, and it was unbearable. We were told to go home on hospice, and that was that. But we still held on to hope, and we didn't listen to them. We were sent on our way later that day, not knowing what was ahead of us, scared out of our minds, and sent home just waiting for him to die. Within a day the blockage cleared and all the swelling in his body went away; it was truly a miracle. Thank God we didn't say anything to the kids and sap more of their childhood away.

We continued the fight for a few weeks, back on the "beat this cancer train" one last time. Unfortunately, it was beating him more than we knew. I woke up at 5 a.m. Wednesday, July 29th, to a big thud. Rob had passed out and fallen in the bathroom. We had nurses check on him during the day, but we didn't know what to think of it. Later that night, we realized that something was going very wrong, and I ended up calling 911. It was terrible. They came in like locusts, so many of them. It was so frightening, especially for the kids. We were taken to the hospital where he was given his final death sentence. It was here. He had another blockage, a blood infection, and cardiac distress. There was nothing that could be done and nothing they could do to save him this time; his body was shutting down. We came home at some ungodly time in the morning and from there begins a blur. Hospice came in, and a bed was delivered. I respected his worst nightmare of setting it up in the dining room and instead had it set up in the room where he sought refuge every day, a room where we could all be and surround him over the next three days. Only three days—it didn't even seem possible. How did it all happen so fast?

From time to time, I can still hear the shrill cries and screams of the kids from when we finally told them and they realized that he was going to die. Rob was able to have a talk with each of them, as much as you can when you know you are not going to be there to see them grow up, graduate from high school, go to college, get married, or hold your first grandchild. How hard it was to listen and realize what was happening; so cruel, so unfair.

By Friday he was already starting to slip into delirium and confusion, at times humoring us with his funny, confused comments. It tore me apart inside to watch him transform into a childlike, almost infantile state. He had always told me he dreaded thinking about that. He was slipping away, and thank God he didn't realize or know because he would have been so embarrassed and horrified at some of the things that happened. To watch him slip away from me, from us, was the hardest thing I have ever witnessed. He was drifting away, reaching for that man with the backpack. Friends, family, and pastors came and went to see him, saying their final goodbyes. Some he looked at and talked to, while others he stared at, not having much recollection that they were there.

By Saturday morning on August 1st, he was totally incoherent. Sadly, I was waiting for him to come to and have one more last final moment of clarity with me, but it never happened. I was lucky to have him talk to me and the kids the day before and hear him tell us how much he loved us and would always be with us no matter what. The day he died was the most peaceful day. Abbie sang and held his hand throughout the day, and a friend came and prayed and sang for him. Later that night our closest friends came, and we all told stories and talked about how he had carried a backpack for someone else so many times, whether while hiking or just the burden of someone's emotional backpack. I shared his vision of the man with the backpack that he saw, and I have to believe that he heard everything we were saying and knew at that point it was time for him to meet that man and go home. Within an hour after they left, he passed away. I was sitting right there next to him on the bed. I had glanced over to say something, and he took his last breath. My mother saw it, and in that moment, she didn't know how she was going to tell me. At that second, she said it seemed like the world just froze. At the same moment, my brother-in-law had a vision while he had drifted off to sleep of what he believed was Rob's spirit leaving us. I turned and just screamed and desperately tried to make it go away and shake him and bring him back. But he was gone, just like that. My partner, my best friend, my body love, gone. Instantly, it was now just me and the kids. It was so much, so much to bear, the cries, the shock, and the reality that he was gone. He lie so still, like a battered wounded soldier who fought so hard and for so long, but finally it was time to surrender.

From there it was a blur, and somehow I made it through the surreal motions of the planning and then experiencing the viewing, the funeral, and the cemetery, now a widow with two young kids. We are on the other side of things, and it is so painful and has left a burning hole in all of our hearts. He fought so hard and rarely ever complained. He was so strong. Through it all he made me strong, enabling me to continue on because of him and my promise to be here for the kids and help them slowly heal.

I know he is there looking after us. I have seen five rainbows in less than six weeks. The first rainbow appeared while we were leaving the cemetery. It was amazing; it looked like an eagle in the sky with a rainbow going right through it and followed us all the way to the reception. The second was our first night at the beach, just two days after the service. He made me promise that, no matter what, I would still go on our planned vacation, and the first night we were there, we looked up in the sky and there was a rainbow. It was just there for us saying, "I'm here, and it's all going to be okay." A couple of nights later, there was a little rain, and Finn was scared, and then after there was the most amazing rainbow we've ever seen. It was as if someone painted the sky with the most beautiful clouds. It was unreal. The fourth one came the night before the kids went back to school, and it was as if he was saying, "I'm here, and good luck tomorrow." And the fifth was almost the most unbelievable. I was walking back from the bus stop in the morning thinking and praying that I was doing a good job with the kids and wondering if he would be proud of me, praying for strength. Then I prayed for a sign, just a small, little sign that he was still here with us, looking and watching, and as I was staring at the sky, a rainbow appeared, just for five seconds or so. It was just for me and then it was gone. I couldn't believe it. I just went into the house and cried, cried from sadness and out of pure joy of having just seen that small, little sign just for me.

Rob was an amazing man, father, husband, son, and friend. He will truly be missed. As we continue to heal and move on throughout the days to come, hopefully we will be blessed with many more rainbows and small signs to know that we will someday be okay until we see him again.

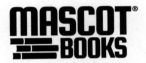

Have a book idea?
Contact us at:
info@mascotbooks.com | www.mascotbooks.com